ISBN-13: 978-1482786316

ISBN-10: 1482786311

SLOW SUICIDE

LIVING WITH DIABETES

and an

EATING DISORDER

Amy Marcle

One of my favorite shows to watch is the new ABC series "Nashville." The other night as I was watching, one of the main characters, "Deacon," made the following statement: "There's thinking about doing something and then there's just doing it." That one line gave me the push I needed to finally do something I have wanted to do for quite some time and that is to write this book.

Writing has always been my passion though few people ever get to read the things I have written. I have always been a very private person mainly because I do not like to put my feelings on the line for fear of getting them crushed. However, this book is by far the most personal piece I have ever written. This is the story of my ongoing battle with Type 1 Diabetes and a deadly eating disorder that almost cost me my life. When I was going through the worst part of my illness, there were not many resources to help me know what normal people dealt with while struggling with this type of problem. I am not writing this to get sympathy, make money, or gain attention. I am writing this to educate and hopefully motivate those who need help to seek it. I hope that by sharing my experiences I can somehow help others who face the same issues.

If you are unaware of just how dangerous eating disorders can be, let me try to help you understand the seriousness of these illnesses. According to the National Institute of Mental Health, eating disorders have the

highest mortality rate of any other mental illness. That fact alone is alarming enough, but add to that the complications of diabetes and you have a deadly combination that is downright terrifying.

Most people are only aware of two types of eating disorders: anorexia and bulimia. While these are the most often recognized, there are many other types of disordered eating behaviors that are just as dangerous. One of the little known disorders being practiced by insulin dependent women is known as diabulimia. Diabulimia is the practice of skipping insulin doses in an attempt to keep blood sugars running way above normal. If the body does not have enough insulin, it will break down fat instead of glucose and use it for energy. When fat is broken down, rapid weight loss occurs, but with a high and deadly price to pay by causing toxins to build up in the blood stream that can lead to coma or death.

Aside from the physical complications that come with an eating disorder, there are so many mental and emotional stresses that are involved it is amazing that anyone can recover. I would dare to say that even though those of us who suffer are overly aware of every ounce we gain or lose, it is not usually our size that is the driving force behind our erratic behavior. The reasons go way beyond wanting to look good in a bathing suit and these reasons vary from person to person. In order to have a successful recovery, it is

necessary that these underlying reasons are identified and treated along with the disorder, and that can sometimes be a difficult task.

As I strive to depict the daily battles I have struggled with, I hope to educate people of this often unnoticed illness that affects many women and men of all ages. My story recaps the diagnosis of my diabetes, what it was like growing up with a long-term illness, and how it affected my life. I will also describe how I almost lost my life to my deadly behaviors and the complications I still face today. If you are looking for an in depth study with a bunch of medical jargon then you have bought the wrong book. However, you will find an honest look into what it's like to suffer with an addiction and how hard it can be to recover. Hopefully, if I can reach just one person and encourage them to get the help they need to get healthy, then my efforts will have been made worthwhile.

WELCOME TO DIABETES

It is obvious that I did not inherit my father's ability to remember dates. My dad, Ernest Pounds, is a retired history teacher and remembers every date of every historical event ever recorded. He can tell you when wars started, when championship games were won, when crimes were committed, and when presidents died. Me? I can barely tell you what today's date is. If it wasn't for Facebook or my cell phone I would not remember anyone's birthday or when I had to be where. There are some dates however I will never forget: that Spring Sunday evening I was baptized, that sad Thanksgiving eve that my Grandmother Laverne died, me and Jason's first date, the day I lost my only grandfather, I knew, and thirteen years later my last living grandmother. I remember, of course, my anniversary and the best day of all, October 29, 2002, the day my daughter was born.

One day I will never forget, even though I wish it had never existed, is December 12, 1990, the day I was diagnosed with Type 1 Diabetes. I had been sick for almost three weeks, well, not really sick, but not really well either. One morning a few weeks prior, I woke up with my skin on fire. My body ached and I was extremely dizzy. I came down the steps for breakfast and spun around in the middle of the kitchen for what seemed an eternity before finally introducing my head to the floor. When I came to, after being passed out cold for a few moments, my parents took me to the doctor. After a few tests and a routine exam, the doctor said I had vasculitis. He explained that it was an inflammation of my blood vessels and that I would feel better in a few days. No worries. And I did feel better, not just in a few days, but only for a few days.

For the nearly four weeks that followed, I stayed extremely exhausted. I was more tired than I had ever been and way more tired than a normal thirteen year old should be. I actually looked forward to naps and going to bed at night. I took naps on weekends. I even started falling asleep in class. I would even take a nap before I could gather up enough energy to climb the steps to my bedroom at night. Also, my appetite changed tremendously. I had never been one to eat many sweet foods, but suddenly I could not get enough sugar to eat. Sugar was the only thing that tasted good. With Christmas just around the corner there were plenty of desserts in the house. One of which was my mom, Kay's, famous homemade fudge. I devoured half a pan of that delicious delicacy one night while the rest of the house was asleep. I should have known then that something was wrong, but, brushed it off as just being a "that time of the month" craving.

More bothersome than my increased desire for the sweet stuff was my intense urge to drink everything I could find within my reach. Tea, coke, juice,

water...you name it I drank it. I not only drank it, but I inhaled it. My thirst was unquenchable and often made me think of what hell might be like. There were many times I found myself in places where having a beverage was not possible and I longed to just dip my tongue in a drop of water to cure my thirst. The real eye-opener for me was when I woke up at 3 am and stumbled down the steps to the refrigerator and grabbed the first thing I could get my hands on. It was not until I had drunk half a gallon that I stopped and took a breath. I had been drinking the one drink that at that time I hated the most....milk. What was wrong with me?

Aside from the cravings and fatigue, was the noticeable weight loss I was experiencing. Nearly thirteen pounds in three weeks. I had never really thought of myself as needing to be on a diet before, but I admit I sure did like the fact that I was eating sugar, drinking sodas, and in the process dropping weight like crazy. Pretty amazing diet plan, I thought to myself. I probably could have enjoyed my newfound weight loss a lot more if I had the energy to put it to use.

Finally, on December 12, 1990, my world came crashing down. I had finished breakfast and was getting ready to go to school like any normal day. That morning, however, was different. I was never the type that wanted to miss school, not because I really wanted to learn, but mainly because I really enjoyed socializing. Today though, I only wanted to visit with my pillow and

a blanket on the couch. I begged my mom to let me skip school and just sleep. Her and my dad had a different idea. It was time to take me to get checked out at the doctor, so to the doctor we went.

If you have ever been to a pediatric clinic, then you know it is not the most peaceful place to be when you already feel like death. I was thirteen at the time and probably the oldest patient at the Children's Clinic that day. I was cranky and those crying, coughing, and screaming toddlers where tap dancing on every nerve in my exhausted body. All I wanted was to be called back into one of those artistically decorated rooms where the tables were covered in white tissue paper and take a nap. I would have waited all day long on Dr. Maley as long as I got to sleep. Sleep and drink. Drink and sleep. Those were my two favorite pastimes.

Dr. Bruce Maley came in and as always made me feel like that even if today was my last day on earth; everything was going to be ok. Dr. Maley was the easiest going person I had ever met. I never minded going to visit him, because being sick was much easier if you had him on your side. He always entered the room with a smile on his face exclaiming "Good Morning Aaammmyy!! How are we today?" But today, he looked concerned. The lab had been testing my blood to see what might be making me feel the way I did, and they discovered pretty quickly the problem. My sugar was unbelievably high. A normal reading was under

100 mg/dl and mine was 383 mg/dl. And then came the diagnosis..."Miss Amy you have what we call Type 1 Diabetes. You will need to be admitted to the hospital for a few days." I sat there stunned. I never showed emotion because that is just not me. Showing emotion opens you up for pain and heartache and I am just not that fond of getting hurt. The nurse came in and instructed my parents on where to take me to be admitted to the hospital. We then proceeded to the patient check out where the receptionist offered me a candy cane for being such a good patient. My mom had already entered her "protective mama bird" zone. "She can't. She has just been diagnosed diabetic." I was in denial and I was mad. I snuck one out in my jacket. "Who knows?" I thought, Dr. Maley and the lab might be wrong.

My mom and dad took me over to the Jackson Madison County Hospital where I was admitted into the Children's Palace, the pediatric wing of the hospital. The hallways were decorated with blue puppy dog prints. I suppose this was done in an attempt to make the children feel better about being in the hospital. After all, who doesn't like little puppies? I can tell you who did not like them at the time...me! I did not like anything or anybody at that very moment. I was greeted by a nurse handing me "Little General", my new stuffed animal puppy friend. I immediately felt out of place. I was the oldest patient on the floor and

nowhere near the sickest. I was wheeled by children much smaller than myself who were facing much bigger battles. Some were facing surgery, others were facing cancer. Each of us was facing different fears, but one thing was certain, we were all scared just the same.

Here it was two weeks before Christmas and I was spending my first night in the hospital ever. My mom stayed with me and though it made me feel good to know she was there, I was still scared. My life had been flipped upside down with the news that I now had a life changing disease that would have to be monitored daily. I was going to be going to classes at the hospital over the next few days to learn how to deal with this new lifestyle. The only thing I had ever heard about diabetes was two things: you could not eat sugar and you had to take shots. I had been craving sugar and I hated shots with a passion. I was also under the impression that the only people who had diabetes were old people. My grandfather had it and I had seen all of those commercials on television with Wilford Brimley talking about his diabetes. Great! Here I was stuck in the kid zone with a disease that only retired folks had. What a life I had to look forward to! That night, after my mom had drifted off to sleep, I did the first thing I had done in a long time. I cried.

For those of you who may be unaware of just what Diabetes is, let me explain. Diabetes is an autoimmune disease in which the pancreas stops producing insulin which regulates the amount of sugar that is in your bloodstream. Too much sugar in the blood stream over time causes damage to all organs in the body. It also affects nerve endings and circulation. It's hard to imagine how one disease can have so many consequences on the body. Once the body stops producing insulin, you have to inject it from an outside source. That's correct. I said inject. This means daily shots, multiple daily shots. I hated shots. I hadn't been diagnosed for 24 hours yet and I already hated the idea of the treatment. But I had no choice. Well actually I did. I could take the shots and live healthy, or I could not take the shots and die. It became pretty obvious which treatment plan I would choose. I mean who would be afraid of something that would save their life? I never dreamed that day would come. But years later, it did.

Aside from learning how much insulin to take and how to do daily sugar checks, I also had to learn how to watch my food intake. I had to learn good foods from bad. Good carbs from not so good carbs. What do you eat? When do you eat? How much do you eat? How often do you eat? Eat...eat...eat. Don't eat! Don't eat! Don't eat! My head was spinning, and my mom was taking notes left and right. How was I ever going to live a normal life with all of these do's and don’ts? Guess I would learn.

One thing I learned while in the hospital was that there are two types of diabetes, the type I have is Type1, also known as Juvenile Diabetes. The other is Type 2 often referred to as adult onset diabetes. Type 2 is caused partly by what you eat and how much you weigh. It can be prevented unlike Type 1. I learned that my diabetes was not anyone's fault. I didn't get it because I ate too much sugar. I was not overweight, so that was not the cause. My body had attacked my own pancreas and caused it to shut down. I burned this information into my brain. I knew I would have to use it later to defend my new illness. I knew that when I got out of the hospital and people found out what I had that they would start asking questions. I wanted to be able to one day tell people that I was not diabetic because I was fat. I was not diabetic because of what I ate. I was diabetic basically because my body got mad at itself and decided it did not want to work anymore. My pancreas had taken an early retirement. While writing this book, I heard a nursing friend of mine put it like this to a patient of his: "Your pancreas took a dump on you!" Thinking about it, I could not have put it better myself. Why was my body attacking itself? Would something else one day decide to just quit working too? I tried to be optimistic and tell myself that it could be much worse. Trying to be positive, I thought to myself, "Ok, here is a battle before me. I can fight it. I can do this." But, my faith in myself and everything else quickly

vanished. I was not as strong as I pretended all those years to be. Being diabetic sucked. Period.

BACK TO NORMAL···IF THAT IS POSSIBLE?

"So, are you going to die? Can I catch your diabetes? If you touch sugar will you die?" These were some of the questions I was bombarded with when I returned to school. This was probably the first time I realized that people know just enough about certain subjects to be dangerous. I was gradually able to get back into a normal routine at school. I had to take breaks during class to check my blood sugar. And, I had to break out peanut butter and crackers every day at 9:15 am to have as a snack. And, I also had to take shots before each meal. Other than those few distractions, life was pretty much normal.

It took some time to get use to what lows and highs felt like. If my sugar dropped too low, I would feel and act funny. Sometimes it would cause me to act down right goofy. Many times when it dropped too low, I would get ill, and at times it would cause me to pass out. My first extreme low happened one day at school. I had not ate much breakfast that morning but had given my normal dose of inulin. Between my first and second classes, I staggered down the hallway to my locker. However, I did not quite make it. The hall started spinning around and around. My eyes were jerking in a fast blink, and my body was shaking. I woke up in the library with my parents and my teachers standing over me. My sugar had plummeted and I had passed out and had a seizure

in the hallway. My head had beaten the floor like a drum and was pounding when I came to my senses. During the seizure, I had bitten my tongue so badly that it remained sore for many days. All I could think about was "what were my friends going to think of me?" I was certain that everyone would stare and point when I went back to school. I did not want to be different.

But, I was different. Up until then, the only noticeable difference between me and anyone else at school was that I was red-headed. Now, I was red-headed and diabetic. I was labeled and though both of those were accurate descriptions of me, I did not want to be branded. Pretty soon I began carrying a chip on my shoulder out of fear that I was being categorized as unhealthy or odd because of my diabetes. I began overthinking every comment that was made to me about my health and began assuming things that were never even said. Because of this, I began feeling the need to make sure everything I did was perfect in an attempt to mask any symptoms that might make people ask questions or pry into my health. Unfortunately, my constant aim to be perfect was setting me up for disaster.

Those of you who know me, know that my father is a minister. And for those of you who are preacher's kids, you know the expectations placed on us. We are sometimes held to a higher standard because we are supposed to be "good" all the time. Those of you who

are preacher's kids are laughing now too because we also get labeled for being the most rebellious. Now take the stress of being held to a higher standard morally and add to that the stress of having to have "perfect" numbers for your weight and your sugar levels and what do you get? In my case, you come up with a teenage girl who became overly obsessed with making sure every single detail of her life was perfect.

First, I became obsessed with numbers. How many carbohydrates did I eat? How many units of insulin did I take? What had my sugar levels been? Count...count...count. Check...check...check. This obsession led to making sure everything was "just right," even things that were not health related. Cords that led from my television had to be lying just right behind the armoire or I couldn't go to sleep. I would check to make sure the curling iron was unplugged over and over and over again before I left the house. I had to check every corner of my bedroom to make sure there were no spiders or stray threads or anything out of place. I didn't realize it at the time, but my brain was becoming programmed to believe that the only way to be happy was to have everything perfect.

It did not help any that the specialist I began seeing was a research doctor who also wanted his patients to be perfect. He was a very knowledgeable doctor whose intentions were probably good, but he lacked the personable skills that I felt a doctor should have. Since

he was a research doctor, every visit made me feel more like a lab rat than a patient. He always came in the exam room with an entourage of residents behind him hanging on his every word like he was a diabetic god. He talked at you and not to you and he was the first person who made me feel hopeless as a diabetic. He prescribed my insulin doses based on my weight. I was to take so many units for ever so many kilograms of weight I carried. At one particular visit, he scolded me for my weight. I had started college and was two pounds heavier than I had been at my prior visit. Two pounds. He instructed me that I really needed to watch my weight and not let it get out of hand. Again, it was only two pounds. I would show him. Boy, would I ever show him! And so it began...my addiction to dieting.

THE COLLEGE YEARS

Criticism has always been one thing I do not handle well even if it is constructive criticism. The lashing I had taken from my doctor had lit a fire under me to prove that I could also make my weight perfect to go along with the "perfect life" I had created for myself. I took the words of my doctor as a challenge. Two pounds. I could lose two pounds, no problem. After all, I was in college. I was taking 18 hours of classes at the University of Tennessee at Martin and was working 35-40 hours a week as night manager at Bradford Bestway. Who had time to eat anyway? I began cutting back on calories and started exercising. When I say cutting back on calories, what I mean is cutting them out, almost all of them out. And when I say I started exercising, I mean excessive exercising. Now that I was on a different schedule every semester, it became easy to hide the fact that I was skipping meals. It became easy to stay up late at night doing aerobics until almost passing out. Breakfast did not exist for me anymore. Lunch was a rice krispy treat and a bottle of water to wash down the diet pills I had started taking. And dinner? A salad...maybe.

Dieting was a challenge at this point because restricting food was causing low blood sugars. In turn, to treat a low blood sugar you have to eat. Eating causes weight gain. The cycle continues over and over and over again.

I was on four insulin injections per day at this time of my life. I learned to adjust my insulin where I could eat less and not get low. My sugars were near perfect and I was losing weight. All was well. I was too busy to notice that I was losing too much weight too quickly.

It wasn't until a friend of mine came up to me at work one day and tried to talk to me about how thin I was looking that I realized I might be headed towards having a serious problem. His exact words were "if you don't start eating, this weekend, instead of us hanging out. I will be attending your funeral." So, I took his advice. I stopped dieting. I began eating normally again and I felt good. I had lost more than the two pounds my doctor had made me feel ashamed of so I felt like I had won. But, there was still more to come. Much more to come.

DATING WITH DIABETES

I'm not a very open person. You have to really earn my trust before I decide to discuss much of anything personal with you. I've always been that way and probably always will. For that reason, I never wanted to tell anyone in high school or college about being diabetic, especially anyone I dated. Looking back, it was stupid for me to be dating someone who knew nothing about my health. I mean, what if I passed out from a low sugar? How would they know what to do? But, at that time I was young and thought I knew everything so I chose not to share my secret with any of my dates.

I can remember one Sunday afternoon when me and the guy I was dating were hanging out at my parents' house. My sugar had been a little off for a few days and I had to check it more often. While we were watching television, my dad and mom asked me if I had checked my sugar. "What? What are you talking about? Check my what?" I desperately tried to make it appear that they were crazy and that I was definitely not diabetic. Looking for a hole to crawl in, I glared at them with that "he doesn't know I'm diabetic" look. I was strongly encouraged to get my tail in the kitchen and check it...NOW! Embarrassed and mad as I had ever been, I went to the kitchen to test my sugar. I then proceeded to tell my date about my diabetes. I quickly

explained that it was NOT because I had been overweight or had eaten too much as a kid. The conversation was awkward to say the least and a few days later the guy called it quits with me. His reason? "I just can't deal with it if I was responsible for you." Wow! Had he really just said that? To my face? While it broke my heart at the time, I learned that sometimes your knight in shining armor turns out to be nothing more than a tin man with no heart.

I had good dating experiences and I had bad, really bad dating experiences before finally meeting Jason. Actually, Jason and I had already met years ago. We worked together in college at Bestway and had known each other for years. We went to high school together, but he was two years behind me in school, so we never really talked to each other. He began working at Bestway with me and we started talking. He had a girlfriend at the time who also worked with us at the store. One night while the "girlfriend" and I were working together, I somehow convinced her that she was too young to be getting serious with Jason and that the only advice I could give her was to suggest that they take a break from each other to decide if they were really right for each other. Jason and I went out shortly after. Think of me what you will, I never said I was always a nice person.

The good thing about Jason was that he knew all about my diabetes. After all, when I had my seizure back in

high school, I had landed on his feet in the hallway. He loves to tell people that he "swept me off my feet." Seriously, it was nice not having to hide my diabetes from him. All of those shots and finger pricks never bothered him at all. His mom, Robbie, is a nurse, so she helped to keep me in check also. Jason and I saw each other at our best and also at our worst. Our personalities were so different; I guess that we somehow balanced each other. We began dating in January 1999 and were engaged that fall. But, there would be one person who would be missing out on our future together. I was about to lose my only grandfather.

LOSING A LOVED ONE

September 1999 was probably one of the hardest months I had experienced to date. My grandfather, Leon Pounds, had been diagnosed with and eventually died from kidney failure caused by, you guessed it, diabetes. He had been a type 2 diabetic for years and like many elderly people with the illness he had, he did not take care of himself like he should have. When he found out his only granddaughter was going to be forced to deal with the more complicated version of the disease he suffered from, he was concerned. At first, he was on oral medication and diet to control his diabetes. Later on, as the medicines stopped being able to control his sugars, he had to take insulin shots. At first, he refused to take them. He told me on many occasions that he did not see how I did it every day and that nobody was going to make him take the daily injections. I was scared for him. I knew what would happen if he did not take his insulin correctly. I knew he would get very sick. I knew he would die. My Granny Jewel, along with the rest of our family, pleaded with him to do the right thing and eventually he did.

However, years of uncontrolled blood sugars on top of his other health conditions did a number on his kidneys. In the last few years of his life, he was forced to take dialysis treatments if he wanted to keep living. Three times a week, every week, he would make the trip to the dialysis clinic where a machine would filter his blood for him since his kidneys could no longer perform the job. Occasionally, I would visit him during his visits. I remember thinking how sad it made me to think that my grandfather and many of the other patients there had to dedicate so much of their time to this process. It really disheartened me because many of them were there due to complications from diabetes.

My grandfather had to follow an even stricter diet than I did since he was in kidney failure. There were good foods. There were bad foods. Foods he could have in limits. Foods he could not have at all. I was starting to realize that when you are diabetic every food becomes either good or bad. There seemed to be no in between. He was also limited on how much liquid he could take in daily. Every time I would visit him, he would have a bowl full of shaved ice that he would be snacking on. I used to fuss at him and tell him that he did not need to be eating so much of it because he was limited on his liquid intake. "It ain't liquid. It's ice!" Bless his heart. Trying to convince him that it would melt was pointless. He even kept little bottles of flavoring in his shirt pocket to make it taste better, more "slushy like" he would say. He often would say that he had lived a good life and he had not been through all he had been through to end up thirsting or starving to death. He would, however, warn me that I needed to always make sure that I took my insulin and do my best to take care of myself. He did

not want me to end up having all of the health problems that he had suffered. I promised him that I would do my best to stay healthy. Although it was unintentional, it ended up being a lie, and a big lie at that.

It did not help any that at the same time my grandfather was battling kidney failure another important person to me was battling cancer. Mr. Ronnie Long, my high school math teacher, had been diagnosed with cancer and was often in and out of the hospital at the same times as Granddaddy. Mr. Long was my favorite teacher in high school. He also came in the store where I worked and we would talk about college and baseball, our favorite sport. We had a rivalry between us because he was a Cardinals fan while I rooted for the Braves. It saddened me to know that two people I enjoyed talking with so much were facing such serious health issues. I knew in the back of my mind that they would end up leaving this world close to the same time. I did not like it, and there was not one thing I could do to prevent it, but I knew it would happen.

In late August 1999, the doctors informed my grandfather and our family that the dialysis treatments were no longer working to filter his blood. By continuing the treatments, he would only be putting his body through unnecessary pain. My grandfather had already told us that when it got to that point, he wanted to stop treatments. He knew that he would only live for

a few days after his final dialysis session, but he was ready. The feelings I had regarding this decision were mixed. I knew that he was tired. I knew that his body was worn out from years of being sick. I also knew that I was selfish. I wanted him to come home and be like he used to be ten years earlier. I wanted to go with him to his garden and pick tomatoes and strawberries. I wanted to play Old Maid and eat Little Debbie's with him again. I wanted to go fishing, sit on the back porch with him, and play with the cats. But, I also wanted him to get the rest he deserved. It helped me to know that he had made his life right with God just months prior to growing sicker. One Sunday, my grandparents visited the congregation where my father preached. During the invitation song, my grandfather came forward to rededicate his life to Christ and to be forgiven for the things he had done wrong. It was the first time in a long time that my eyes had gotten teary. I was proud of him and I was glad that I was there to see him show this courage. Finally, I was able to accept the fact that we only had a few more days left to visit with him. Though, I was still deeply saddened losing him, I decided to make the most of each day I had left with him.

Granddaddy had always enjoyed being at home. He loved it when anybody would come visit him and my grandmother. When I would go see them, it did not matter if I stayed five minutes or five hours, when I got

ready to leave he always said the same thing..."what's your hurry? You just got here!" Even though Granddaddy loved home so much, he had made it clear he did not want to die there. He thought it would be too hard on my grandmother. The last ten days of his life were spent in the hospital. We visited everyday even though the last couple of days he was pretty much unresponsive. My parents, my brother and his family, Jason, and I would sit in the hall and take turns going in to check on him. There was this particular day where we had been there all day and I was growing tired both physically and emotionally. It was getting close to 5:00 pm and I had asked Jason to drive me home. I went in to tell Granddaddy that I was leaving and that I would see him the next day. When I leaned in to kiss his forehead, he opened his eyes and said "where you going? You just got here!" I could not help but laugh as I told him I had been there all day but that he had been napping for the biggest part of the afternoon. He nodded his head and drifted back to sleep. That was the last conversation I had with him.

When Jason and I arrived at his parent's house that same night, Jason's mom told us that Mr. Long had passed away that afternoon. The first part of my prediction had become reality. He had been in the hospital while my grandfather was there. My father had gone to see him and cautioned me not to visit him.

He told me that I should remember him the way I had always known him. Healthy and happy.

I went home that night and sat up talking to my Mom for a long time. Dad was staying at the hospital that evening to keep my grandmother company. My grandfather had made my dad promise to take care of her when he died, and my father did not want her being there alone in case something happened during the night. My house phone rang around 2 am. It was my father calling to ask my mom to come to the hospital. My grandfather had gotten much worse. Within an hour, I got the call that he had passed away. As I had predicted, him and Mr. Long had left their pain behind less than twelve hours apart.

While I was sad, I was also relieved. The pain that Granddaddy had was no longer an issue. He had gone to a much better place than we were. I did feel regrets for never fulfilling the promise I made to him. He had to miss my college graduation due to his illness, and I had promised him that I would bring the video over and we would watch it together. I never got around to doing that and I thought of that during the visitation. I went home that night and wrote the following poem about him. I think he would have been proud.

GRANDADDY

Today we meet in honor

Of you who's now at rest

To remember how you lived your life

To its fullest and its best

We remember all the happiness

You helped to provide

And how when you were needed

You were right there at our side

We remember how you

Cared about others like you did

And how the love you had for your family

Was never from us kept hid

We remember you as a husband and father

Who was there to hold our hand

And as wonderful grandfather

To the children great and grand

We remember all the pain

That in your life you faced

But are thankful that you now have a home

In that beautiful resting place

Slow Suicide

So we cry not out of sorrow

Though we know how it does hurt

We cry because we're happy

You now have the rest and peace you so deserve.

GETTING HITCHED

After I graduated from college, I continued to work at Bestway because I had yet to find another job that I thought would suit me. In December 1999, I was hired at Porter Cable as a marketing assistant to the product development team. It was a decent job and, of course, paid more than I had been making at the grocery store. But, it wasn't me. I had a cubicle that I worked from and everyday reminded me of the movie "Office Space." From my boss asking me about crazy reports down to the copy machine I wanted to take to a field and beat with a baseball bat, it was just like the movie. After I had been there about six months, rumors began to circulate about a potential huge layoff. I had already suspected that our emails were being monitored, so I began sending out emails to friends outside of the company expressing how much I disliked my new job. I was used to being around people all the time at the store and sitting in a cubicle was just not cutting it for me. Within two weeks I was called into my boss's office and informed that due to a decrease in sales and increased costs in production my position was one of many that was being cut. I was not the only one let go that day, but I was probably the only one who was happy about it. I wanted to be back in an environment where I could socialize with customers and co-workers. I wanted to be back in the grocery business.

The layoff did come at somewhat of a bad time. It was late July 2000 and Jason and I were engaged to be married in November of that year. Here it was four months before the wedding and I was out of a job. I contacted a former manager of mine to see if he knew of any job openings in the grocery business. In early September, he called to tell me of a position opened with Food Rite in Dyer. I interviewed and began working for them on September 5, 2000. Now we could go ahead as planned with our wedding. There was only one slight problem. I still had not told my parents that we had set a date.

We had put down a deposit at The Primrose House in Medina for November. Jason kept telling me that I had to tell my parents or else they would be upset with us. I am not really sure why I kept putting it off. Perhaps I was afraid to leave home, afraid of becoming homesick, or scared to move forward in my life. Whatever the reason was, I could not make myself tell them. We had to lose the deposit at the wedding chapel we were going to use and we reset the date for December 9th. I waited until less than 6 weeks before the wedding to inform my parents of the date. I know they were hurt. They were also concerned. "Where do you think you are going to find a place to live on this short of a notice?" they asked. It was then that I told them we had just closed on a house in Milan. After some pretty intense conversations about how disrespectful I had been, we

began the wedding planning process. Looking back I think it was better that we had less time to plan. Less time to plan meant less time to stress.

Finally, the big day arrived. We had a morning wedding so that we could get to Gatlinburg by early evening. We were still able to have the ceremony at The Primrose House. They took care of everything except for the flowers, photos, and cake. When we arrived that morning everything looked amazing! However, with all of the running around and hurrying to get ready, my diabetes decided to show out and my sugar crashed. Great! Here it was one hour before I was to walk down a hardwood staircase in three inch heels and I could barely even stand up. Luckily, my photographer brought me punch and mints from the reception area. I am probably one of the only brides who went to the reception before the wedding! Nauseas and now on a sugar high, I managed to feel better just in time to walk down the aisle. To this day when Jason's friends ask me "what made you marry him?" many times I tell them that my sugar was low that day and that I was unaware of anything that was happening.

Being that my father was the only minister I had ever really known, we asked him to perform the ceremony. My brother, Allen, walked me down the aisle and gave me away. My mom, bless her heart, held it together as she watched the love of her life perform the wedding ceremony of her only daughter who was being given away by her only son. My father managed to do very well. I only saw his lip quiver once.

After the ceremony, the reception, and all of the pictures, the gentleman who owned the Primrose House came and asked if he could speak with me. He took me into a side room and told me that he had heard I was diabetic and had gotten low that morning. He asked if I felt better and if I needed anything to take with me for the trip to East Tennessee. He then shared a part of his life with me that was very touching and personal. His son was also diabetic and took insulin. One day when he was on his way home, his sugar dropped as he was driving. He passed out and his car ran off the road and caught fire. Sadly, his son died in the accident. He told me he wanted to share that with me because he wanted me to take care of myself. He asked me to promise him that I would always check my sugar before I dared to drive a car. I thanked him for the story and promised him I would. Again, another unintentional lie

After the honeymoon, Jason and I returned to our home In Milan and started getting adjusted to our new life. He worked in Jackson and I was working in Dyer, so making our home in Milan helped to split the difference in our travel. Soon after we were married, I was offered the bookkeeping job at Food Rite's Dyer store. I had been traveling to the other stores to oversee the Health and Beauty Aid departments. This new job

meant that I would not have to travel between stores anymore which was about to come in very handy.

Sugar for Two

Jason and I had been married for fourteen months when we received the best news we could have ever gotten...we were going to have a baby! It was February 2002, and our newest addition was due in November, just in time for a special holiday season. While we were excited, we knew that I would have to take extra precautions to guarantee a healthy delivery. I was going to have to keep my blood sugar at near perfect levels to keep our child from having birth defects. Knowing that high blood sugars can cause many problems for both the mother and the baby, I knew it was crucial that I took very good care of myself.

Because of my diabetes, I was considered a high risk case and instead of the monthly doctor visits that most expecting mothers have, I made weekly trips to my doctor. The reason for the weekly visits was to adjust my insulin to keep my blood sugars in balance. I was dedicated to keeping them near perfect. Matter of fact, they never ran high during the entire nine months. Instead, they stayed low, dangerously low. The low blood sugars were a cause for worry for my family. They were afraid to leave me alone for long periods of time because they feared I would have a low sugar episode and slip into a diabetic coma. Unfortunately, their fears came true over and over again.

The first scary episode came just eight weeks into my pregnancy. I was at work and suddenly got to feeling dizzy. I was on my way to the restroom and convinced myself that I would be fine to wait until I was out of the restroom to check my blood sugar. Wrong! After being missing in action for close to 45 minutes, my co-workers began questioning my whereabouts. Someone had heard screams coming from the backroom but brushed them off as someone just goofing off. Again someone asked where I was as they again heard screaming from the locked bathroom. My friend and store manager, Tonya King, kicked in the door to find me passed out cold and half naked on the bathroom floor.

When I came to, I found myself surrounded by co-workers and paramedics. The first thought that ran through my head was "is my baby ok?" followed by "why am I wearing a meat smock as a wrap skirt?" The only thing I could remember was I believed that the bathroom was a dungeon and that I had been trapped inside. I looked at my fingers and my nails were bleeding from where I had tried to claw my way out through the tile floor. I had no clue where I was or why I was laying on a stretcher. My sugar had bottomed out and was so low that it would not even register on the glucose monitor. Tonya and Brenda Oliver had tried their best to get me dressed, but my skin was so clammy that they had to just wrap me in a meat jacket instead. The paramedics gave me a shot of glucagon to raise my

sugar and then quickly transported me to the hospital. Jason met me at the emergency room where they ran tests and performed ultrasounds to reassure me that my baby had not suffered any trauma. I stayed a few hours for observation before finally being released. The next day I returned to work dreading to face the embarrassment of being found half clothed in the restroom. After everyone was certain that both my baby and I were going to be ok, the jokes began. "You been in any dungeons lately?" and "Gonna show your butt today, Amy?" were just a few of the jokes I had to endure. One of my co-workers was attending EMT school at the time. He informed me that he started to come help me, but when he heard I was laid out "sunny side up" he was afraid it would make for an uncomfortable situation when I got back to work. I told him I was glad to know that if my house caught on fire while I was in the shower, he would just let me burn up and die rather than save my life and then feel uncomfortable afterwards! Seriously, it was a very scary situation at the time, but I learned that I was going to have to learn to laugh at myself because more episodes were to follow. For the rest of my pregnancy, I had to report in before going to the restroom, just to be safe. They had even decided to nickname my unborn child "Lo Lo" since my sugar stayed low so much. Bless her heart; she kept that nickname until the day she was born.

The next scary incident came on a Sunday afternoon. Jason and I had come home from church and were just having a lazy day. All of a sudden, Jason told me he thought I needed to go check my sugar because I was acting weird. I had been diabetic so long and had heard that so much that I had grown tired of hearing people tell me to "check your sugar." I insisted that I was fine and went on doing whatever it was I was doing. Later, I got up and started stumbling into the walls and knocking pictures off the tables as I fell. Jason again insisted that I needed to check my sugar. His demands did not set well with me. I was low, there was no denying it. But, I was also mad now. I had been eating some of those goldfish cheesy crackers and like a two year old, I took and poured the entire box all over our bed. I climbed on the bed and starting jumping up and down on the crackers, grinding them into a fine powder with my bare feet until all that could be seen was a room filled with an orange, cheesy fog.

Jason's dad, Danny, had stopped by and the two of them tried their best to calm me down and get me to eat something. Jason picked me up and carried me, kicking and screaming, into the kitchen. He was trying to help me, but I thought he was trying to kill me. I began hitting him and even slapped him in the face, demanding that he put me down. "I swear I will call the police and tell them you are assaulting me!" I screamed. They attempted to put sugar under my tongue to help

raise my glucose only to have me spit it back in their face. They were finally able to hold me down and inject me with glucagon. After a few moments, I began to feel better and then upset at the mess I had made. Cheese dust everywhere! Broken glass. Stuff scattered. "You were mean!" Jason told me. He told me everything that I had done and I could not believe that I had acted in such a way. That's what happens when my sugar gets out of whack. I become a completely different person and usually remember very little.

Perhaps the scariest moment, during the entire nine months, came when I was eight months pregnant. I had seen so many close calls and "near misses" during the last few months that people were scared to leave me alone. I had passed out more times than I could count. But, I was still independent and still drove to work every day. That freedom would soon come to an abrupt end.

I was on my way home from work one afternoon and decided to call my mother just to chat. As we talked, she began to question me. "What's your sugar? Where are you? You sound weird. You need to pull over." I assured her that I was fine and that I would check it when I got home. After all, I was only 15 minutes away from my house. I continued to drive and made it to my house, but I did not stop. Jason was in the driveway waving frantically in an attempt to get me to slow down. My mom had called him and told him she thought I was

driving with low sugar. They had tried to call my cell phone, but I was so unaware of where I was that I did not answer.

I drove past my house and waved at Jason. I had no clue who he was. I just thought it was nice of that sweet fellow to be waving like that at the cars passing his yard. I travelled onward. I crossed a set of railroad tracks and finally stopped when I ran off the road and hit a telephone pole. I did not have to wait for the cops to arrive. They had been chasing me since I had left Trenton. Someone had called central control to report a possible drunk driver on the Milan-Trenton Highway. I definitely was not drunk. The thing about low blood sugar is that it can make you appear to be completely intoxicated without having ever touched alcohol. My cell phone was ringing in the passenger seat and one of the police officers answered. It was Jason. He told them not to arrest me that I was not drunk and informed them of my condition. They called the paramedics and I was transported to the hospital AGAIN to get checked out. Thankfully, Haley was unharmed and all I had were multiple bruises across the forehead and face where my head had banged into the steering wheel. It had to have been the protective hand of God who drove me home that day. I had driven nearly twelve miles almost completely unconscious. All it would have taken was a train on that track. A curve missed. Another car stopping in front of me. Any of

those, and I would have not been here today to write about it. Even worse, I would not have had the beautiful daughter I have today.

After my wreck, the doctors, along with the Milan police department, put me on driving probation. I was not allowed to drive again until after Haley was to be born. So, my parents took turns shuttling me back and forth to work each day. I hated being dependent on them or anyone else. I was and still am a very stubborn, independent person. My pleadings to allow me to drive were voted down. Safety had to be put ahead of my pride for the sake of my child and, at the time, any driver on the road.

On October 25th, I called my doctor's office to schedule an appointment. I was 39 weeks along and ready to see my bundle of joy. My doctors had already told me that they would not let me go past 39 weeks to prevent having any problems. When the receptionist answered, she asked if I was calling to schedule a regular appointment or was something wrong. "No," I replied, "I am calling to schedule an inducement of labor. I was told I would not have to go past 39 weeks in labor by my doctor, and today I am exactly 39 weeks! See if you can't get me in for Monday morning." After a brief pause, she came back and said to be at the hospital on Monday to have my labor induced. Finally, we were getting close to our big day!

Monday came and I was extremely nervous and excited. We met with the admissions department where the lady, never looking up from her computer, asked why I was there. I looked at Jason and then at my overly pregnant tummy. I could barely contain my desire to use sarcasm and started to tell her I was there for a breast reduction, but I decided against it and told here I was having a baby. We were escorted upstairs to the maternity department. Boy! That place was hopping that morning! Pregnant women and nervous dads to be everywhere! We later heard that there were 23 babies born that day. However, not one of those newborns was our little Haley. She was playing the waiting game. And she was good at it. My last ultrasound had showed her looking rather comfortable and well entertained as she was using her tiny little hands to flick the umbilical cord back and forth. I guess she was playing in there and having such a good time that she was not quite ready to come out. It was also my nephew's birthday and I suppose she felt she wanted to have her own special day. She wanted to stand out and boy does she do that well! So, we waited. I was growing uncomfortable and very irritable. Jason was making me so mad that if I could have gotten out of the hospital bed I would have probably inflicted him with bodily harm. A contraction would hit and I would grumble about being in pain and he would say, "Well, why are you hurting?" Gee! I could not imagine why I was hurting. I mean after all, here I was a living breathing

human attempting to have another live human slowly crawl out of my body. I called Jason names in front of my mother that she probably never dreamed I would say. What's worse than cussing your husband in front of your mom? Finding out later that your preacher was outside the door and heard the whole thing! My mother-in-law finally convinced Jason it would be best for him to go find him some coffee and give me a little space.

The staff was great even though I was not the best patient. I already knew that I was going to accept all of the pain medicine they would allow me to have before, during, and after the delivery. There was no way I could be one of those moms who would one day brag about having their baby naturally. I wasn't there for bragging rights on my delivery. I was there to brag about the beautiful baby I was going to be taking home with me. I kept asking when I would be able to have my epidural. When they finally brought it in to administer it to me, the nurse informed me that she was surprised they were just now allowing me to have it. "You mean I could have had this an hour ago??!!??" I questioned. "Are you kidding me?" I looked at my sweet little nurse who looked to be about six months pregnant herself. "Oh my word! You are having one too! I am so sorry for making it appear that this is not fun. It's really not that bad." I was trying hard to smooth things over and not make her dread her own experience that

she was going to be having in the near future. She laughed and reassured me that she had seen much worse patients than me. After the pain subsided, I was able to drift off to sleep. It's unclear who enjoyed my nap the most, me or the staff and my family who were just glad for me to be quiet for a few hours.

Finally at 7:21 pm on Tuesday, October 29th, Haley Brooke Marcle made her grand entrance into this world. It still was not by her choice, but both of our heart rates were starting to get too fast, and Dr. Wilson advised me to have a C-section. It was going to be too much of a risk to continue to wait on her to arrive on her own. I agreed, and within a few moments, I heard her crying.

Hearing her cry for the first time was the most beautiful sound I had ever heard. She was perfect. Perfect little round head. Perfect little toes. Perfect little fingers. All of the hard times I had experienced during pregnancy faded away when I saw her. She was definitely worth the nine month wait. Definitely worth the high and low blood sugars, the mood swings, the diabetic comas, and the car accident. Haley was taken to the neo-natal unit right after her birth. She had...you guessed it...low blood sugar. Her glucose registered at 23 mg/dl. The nurses and doctors assured me that this was normal for babies of diabetic mothers and that she would be fine. She spent her first night in the NICU so she could be monitored and so I could rest. Rest was

out of the question. Though I was told that she would be fine, I worried that she was going to inherit my blood sugar problems. Thankfully, my worries never became reality. The next day we got to have her in our room with us. We went home two days after she was born which was on Halloween. The absolute best treat ever!

Settling In

The three of us were able to settle into our new life at home fairly quickly. Jason took off a week from work so he could spend some time with us. After he returned to work, Haley and I really enjoyed bonding with each other. Well, I enjoyed it, she mostly slept. We spent our mornings watching Andy Griffith and Dick Van Dyke. I also introduced her to country music by rocking her to the tunes of the videos playing on CMT. When she slept, I slept. When she cried, I admit I cried too. Exhausted does not begin to describe how tired I was during that time. But, I was completely in awe of her. I was also afraid that I would mess up and do something wrong. So, I kept a check on her constantly. Jason had to keep reassuring me that I did not have to feel of her every time she fell asleep to make sure she was still breathing. But, I could not help myself. I had to make sure she was ok. She never slept in her crib. Never. Not one single night. Her crib became a stuffed animal habitat instead. When she slept, it was on my chest. People told me that I was spoiling her by holding her so much and that one day I would "pay for it." All of the unsolicited advice on parenting angered me and I blew off those comments, thinking that she was my child and she would only be little for a short time. If I wanted to hold her, then I was going to hold her. And if by "paying for it," those people meant that we would one day have the bond that she and I share today, then I

am definitely paying for it and enjoying every moment of it.

I never really thought about the weight I had gained during pregnancy until it was getting close to time to return to work. Suddenly, I realized that it was time to get in shape. I had lost some of the weight I had put on, but was nowhere near where I wanted to be. I began eating right and cutting back on the junk food I had ate during my maternity leave. Hopefully, when I got back to work I would get back to a healthy eating pattern. Hopefully, the weight would start to come off. And it did, but at an unbelievable price.

The Danger Begins

Going back to work was hard for me. Like all new mothers, I was reluctant to leave my baby. My mom kept Haley for the first two weeks while we waited on a spot to open up at daycare. There was a daycare across the street from the store and we were waiting to get Haley in there. Having her so close made it much easier to leave her each day.

I was, however, getting discouraged about not being able to lose the last ten pounds I needed to in order to get back to my pre-pregnancy weight. My blood sugar was also beginning to stay high due to lack of sleep and the everyday stress that comes with being a new mom. But one thing I did notice was that when my sugar was high, I was not hungry. Not hungry at all. As I thought about that, I was reminded of how quickly I lost weight when I first found out about my diabetes. My sugars had been high then and I had dropped weight like crazy. You could almost see the light bulb pop on over my head. If I could manage to keep my sugar just high enough to burn the weight off, then I could drop these last few pounds. And so it began, I was entering the dangerous and deadly world of "diabulimia."

I started out by just cutting my insulin back a few units per shot. I did not want to get sick after all, I just wanted to run slightly high for just a couple of weeks.

My sugars started staying between 200 and 250 mg/dl. These levels were high, but nowhere near high enough to cause me to lose the weight fast enough. At that time, I was giving four insulin shots a day. I took it upon myself to cut out one of those. I also began drinking sodas with sugar in them in an attempt to run my levels up that much more. It was working. Little by little I was losing the weight I had wanted to get rid of so badly.

The people at work had gotten so use to making me check my sugar while I was pregnant that they kept doing so afterwards. When some of them noticed it was running high, they began to get concerned. "And you're losing weight too. And you're losing it quick. Is it because your sugar is high? "Tonya asked me one day. What? No! No way! It's just a coincidence. That was all. I was beginning to cover my secret with lies. The first of many, many lies.

If cutting out one insulin shot was working, then cutting out two would work even better. That was the reasoning inside my head. Then I could get this over with much quicker and get back to normal. Little did I know at that time that there would never be any getting back to normal.

I was tired and extremely thirsty all the time, classic symptoms for an out of control diabetic. I would come home from work and fall asleep as soon as I hit the

couch or recliner. Jason became very frustrated because I would even fall asleep as he was talking to me. He would question me about my sugars. Was it high? The lies came easy. No. It was good. When he would ask me what it was I would just pull a number out of the air and tell him that's what it was. How was I to know? I would sometimes go days without even checking it.

My dangerous habits went on for about two months before things got really bad. And really bad is putting it mildly.

Skipping just one shot here and there was not enough, so I pushed myself into going a few days at a time without injecting my life saving meds. My body was growing use to the "high" feeling that I was experiencing from outrageously elevated sugar levels. Feeling bad began to feel good. I was beginning to act just like a drug addict. I was addicted to the way I felt when truthfully I felt horribly sick. I could not dwell on that at the time, I had weight I had to lose and so far this was the easiest plan ever. It never occurred to me that I was headed down a deadly path until it was almost too late.

FEBRUARY 12, 2003

My deadly diet tricks were beginning to catch up with me. I had lost all of the weight I had set out to lose, but just could not stop restricting my insulin. What if I gave it and gained back what I had lost? I did not trust it anymore. It did not matter that insulin was the only thing that would keep me alive. It was also going to keep me from losing weight , and I was not about to become a failure and gain back any of the weight I had worked so hard to lose.

Down 15 pounds in three weeks, I was proud of my success, even though I did not have the energy to enjoy my weight loss. Finally, on February 12, 2003, my lies and secrets caught up with me as my life almost came to an end.

I got up that morning and got ready for work and had also gotten Haley ready for daycare. She was only four months old at the time, and was just getting over RSV. Needless to say it had been several nights since either of us had slept well and again I was worn out. I drove to Dyer and stopped by my friend, Tonya's, house. She lives next to the store and close to Haley's daycare. I asked her if she could drive me the tenth of a mile to the daycare and help me get Haley out of the car. I was just too weak to do it by myself. She tried to get me to call Jason or my parents to have them take me to the doctor,

but, I refused. I just needed to rest. Just like the day I was diagnosed, I convinced myself that a short nap was all I needed. Much like a hangover, I just needed to sleep it off.

After getting Haley checked in at daycare, I went to work. I looked horrible. I felt horrible. My sugar was so high that I could barely function. I was so dehydrated that my eyes were dried out and burning. I was so exhausted that I could barely hold my head up. I asked Tonya if she would let me go to her house to take a nap. I would come back in an hour and use this as my lunch break if they would let me; I just had to get some sleep. She agreed and I went to take a nap on her couch. While I was gone, she called a friend of hers who was a nurse practitioner. She told her how I was acting and what I looked like. Her friend told her that I needed to get to a doctor ASAP. She called a physician in Trenton and made me an appointment for that afternoon. I was reluctant to go, but I did not have the strength to argue with her. I finally agreed to go if she would just let me sleep until it was time for me to drag myself off of the couch and go see what was going on with me. I did not dare want to tell anyone what I had been doing at that time. They would find out soon enough. I called Jason and told him I was going to the doctor and that Tonya was going to drive me. I insisted that I would be fine and that I just wanted to get checked out. I promised to call him when I was done.

My body ached and my skin was so flushed and feverish that it hurt to even touch my cheek. I had been nibbling on ice because of the intense thirst I was experiencing. But, even bites of ice were making me nauseas. Sleep was what I was craving. Just one more little nap and then I would be fine. I had even started to believe my own lies , trying desperately not to see that my self-induced illness was going to be the death of me.

When I arrived at the doctor's office, they began to run a series of blood tests. I was beginning to feel very sick and irritable at this time and really just wanted to lie down. When the doctor entered the exam room, he told me that my sugar was high. Dangerously high. He informed me that I was in diabetic ketoacidosis. I knew what that meant. I had experienced that during my initial diagnosis too. For a diabetic, this was definitely not good news.

Diabetic ketoacidosis (DKA) is when your body does not get the glucose it needs for energy; it begins to burn fat for energy instead. This is why you lose weight quickly when your sugar is high. When fat is burned for energy, ketones are produced in the blood and appear in the urine when you do not have enough insulin. When ketones show up in a urinalysis, it is a sign that the diabetes is out of control and that severe sickness is about to follow. High levels of these ketones can be poison to the body and thus leads to DKA. DKA also causes the body's electrolytes such as sodium,

potassium, and chloride to be depleted making you that much sicker. If left untreated, DKA can lead to loss of consciousness and even death.

The doctor told me to get to the hospital in Jackson as soon as possible. Do not stop. Do not go home. Leave. Leave now. I called Jason and told him I was heading to the hospital and for him to meet me at the E.R. Tonya drove me there. I was too weak to call my parents, so she had to call them for me and let them know what was going on with me. My mom went to pick up Haley while my dad met me at the hospital. Thinking back, I am not sure which I was more afraid of, informing them of my desperate attempts to lose weight or knowing that I was going to have to put my weight loss on the back burner for a few days.

Though I felt like crying, I did not shed the first tear. There was not enough fluid in my body to produce tears anyway. I was scared. I was scared of what I had done to my body. I was scared I would get very sick. I was scared I would die. Knowing that I was about to be hospitalized for something I had brought upon myself, I knew that I was going to have to admit the reasons for my sugar being high. I knew nobody would understand my motives. Nobody even understood what it was like to be diabetic. At least, nobody that I was close to did. I admitted to Tonya that I had been keeping my sugar high to lose weight. I was afraid to tell Jason. I was

afraid he would be mad at me. Maybe I was just afraid he would make me stop.

We arrived at the emergency room and I immediately ran to the restroom to throw up. My breathing was labored as a result of my blood being acidic. My lungs were working overtime to blow the acid out of my body. Worried and frightened, I asked Tonya if I was going to die. She did not dare to answer, because at that moment my future was uncertain.

I was taken back to an observation room where Jason soon met me along with my father. Again, I began throwing up on the table. My breathing was worse, much worse, and the E.R. staffed debated my need for oxygen. I asked Jason were Haley was, scared that I might not see her again. My dad informed me that she was with my mom and was doing fine. I really could not remember if I had picked her up that day or even how I had gotten to the hospital. Doctors and nurses were scurrying around me on all sides, drawing blood, and performing tests. Bags of IV fluids were hanging above my head and draining into my veins in a desperate attempt to keep me alive.

I woke up six hours later in the intensive care unit. My mouth was parched due to severe dehydration. There was a bright light shining over me and for a moment I thought I was dead. Little did I know that had almost been my fate. When I was finally able to open my eyes,

I saw Jason and my father-in-law standing over me. Jason told me that I had gotten very sick from my blood sugar being so high. He told me that I was in the intensive care unit and that they could only visit me for a few minutes. He let me know that Haley was with my parents and that she was ok. They were uncertain why my sugar had been so elevated but they were doing everything necessary to bring it back to a normal level. I wanted to tell him why I was so sick, but I was just so tired and so confused and too weak to talk. I begged for something to drink but was only allowed a few ice chips. They had to leave soon. Jason promised he would be downstairs in the family waiting room and would stay there all night. The nurse came in and told them visiting hours were over and I was left alone in the dark. Frightened, but too drained to really care.

When I woke up the next morning, I was still baffled. I could not remember why I was in ICU. Where was everyone? Why was I here? I looked around at the tubes and monitors hooked up to my body. There were bags of IV fluids hanging and pumping me full of electrolytes I had lost. I was wearing a heart monitor and an oxygen monitor. Insulin was dripping into my veins at a slow, steady rate. My arms were battered and bruised from the many blood tests they had done in the emergency room.

At 9:00 am, Jason came in to visit. He sat down and explained to me what had happened. He did not know

why yet. He only knew that my sugar had gotten out of control and that was the reason I had gotten so sick. Then he told me the following: "The emergency room doctor said you were very lucky. He pulled me outside last night and told me that you almost did not make it. Your breathing and heart rate were so bad that had you been thirty minutes later getting to the hospital you would have died." I tried to let that sink in. Thirty minutes? Jason put it in perspective for me. "If you had gotten stuck in traffic, if your appointment in Trenton had been later, if you had gotten stopped by a cop or by a train then you would not be here." I asked him if he was sure that is what the doctor said. I made him repeat it to me over and over and over again. How could I have been so stupid? How could I have put my life at risk to lose those extra pounds? I confessed to Jason what I had done. I also later told my parents. I believe we were all in denial and probably in shock that I would do something so drastic. I swore to never do it again. I just wanted to go home. I wanted to be with Haley and be healthy again.

I spent five days in ICU. My electrolytes were so out of line that it took that long to get them back where they should be. One of the main concerns was my potassium was still way too low and had to be corrected to prevent any type of negative effects to my heart My blood's pH level was also out of balance. The body tries to maintain a pH level of 7.4 as a neutral state. Anything less than 6.9 means the blood is acidic. My level was right at 4.0. Basically, my blood was like acid running through my veins. I endured hourly sugar checks and more intensive labs every four hours. I had the absolute best nurse ever, a gentleman who not only did his best to take care of me, but also let my family "bend the rules" and stay with me longer during the visits. He even talked to me about how dangerous my diet had become. When I left the intensive care unit, I wanted to take him with me for moral support. I was hungry too. I had not eaten real food in several days. After what I had put my body through, the hunger was setting in and I was literally starving.

Finally, I was allowed to go to a regular patient room. Soon, I would be allowed to see Haley again. My family brought her to visit me and it seemed that she had grown bushels in those five days. I was afraid that she had forgotten me. She cried and screamed when I tried to hold her. It broke my heart to see her afraid of the tubes running out of my arms. I was ready to be back to normal. I stayed another night and then was discharged. I was given a new sliding scale for my insulin shots and a diet plan to make sure I received the right amount of nutrients. The doctors were not aware that my high sugars were intentional. I swore I would follow these new rules. Again, I lied.

From Bad to Worse

The bad thing about losing weight so quickly is that you gain it back and then some just as fast if not faster than you lost it. I was badly dehydrated when I entered the hospital. I went through what seemed like hundreds of bags of fluids to help get me back to where I needed to be. With all of those fluids going through me in such a short amount of time, I ballooned up quickly. I kept trying to be positive, thinking that the weight I had gained back was just from retaining fluids and hoped it would disappear in just a few days. Unfortunately, I am not a very patient person. Within a few days, I was already planning ways to lose back down. Water or not…I DID NOT want it on my body. Period.

I knew that I was under constant surveillance since my near death episode a few weeks earlier. Everyone was watching my every move. "Did you take you insulin? Did you check your sugar? Are you high? Are you low? Did you eat?" Everywhere I turned I was being watched and questioned like a criminal. I can't say that I blame my family and friends. After all, with what I had done, I would not trust me either. I was going to have to get sneaky if I was going to lose weight now. I was definitely going to have to step up my game.

Within a week after leaving the hospital, I slowly began cutting back my insulin again. I did not want to do

anything too drastic right off the bat. I had to work slower this time if I wanted to sneak my habits by the onlookers. Though I had gotten good at lying earlier about what my sugars were, lying seemed to be getting easier with each story I told. I had quit checking my sugars. I knew they were high, so there was no point wasting test strips to find this out. Plus, it really did not matter what the meter said, I was not going to give anything to help lower it anyway. I was starting to get tired all the time, so I knew the diet was working. I knew that being tired, thirsty, and irritable were signs that my sugar was running high. Knowing that being in DKA was a sure fire way to burn off extra calories, I bought test strips to determine if I was passing ketones. I could check this at home and know for sure if I was getting close to entering the danger zone again. If I could keep them high enough to show up but low enough to stay out of the hospital, then I could have the best of both worlds. Most diabetics check their ketones to prevent DKA, but I was checking them to guarantee that I was in DKA so the fat would start coming off. And it did…quickly.

Within just a few months, I was back in the hospital again. I had done a pretty good job of covering the fact that my sugars were running between 300 and 400 mg/dl on a daily basis. I slept with my monitor under my pillow so Jason would not find it and be able to see that I had not checked it in days. And of course, when

asked what they had been running, I lied. Somehow I had gained Jason and my parents' trust again so when I began being admitted to the hospital so often; they began wondering why I was so sick. Why was I in DKA again? Why was the insulin not working? This went on for weeks and weeks. I pretended to be in just as much shock as the doctors and my family was. What was the plan to make my insulin work correctly? Oh, that's right…maybe actually taking it would help. Instead of confessing to restricting my insulin, I allowed the doctors to scratch their heads as they tried to determine what my next course of treatment should be. Again, I was pumped with fluids, given a new sliding scale of how much insulin to take, and sent home. The doctors would suggest following up in a few weeks, but I refused. Keeping appointments meant the doctor would expect me to get my sugar under control. But, if I failed to follow up, then nobody would catch on to my deadly secret. So, I changed doctors like most people change out their toothbrush, every few weeks. Never keep the same doctor when you have something to hide, I had learned. Never!

I began reasoning in my head that if one dangerous trick to lose weight would work, then adding more tricks would make me even skinnier. I started restricting the amount of calories I consumed in a day. I had to watch how I handled this since everyone was watching that too. When I skipped dinner, I would tell

Jason I ate in the other room already, or that I had a big lunch. I would sometimes tell him I was just too tired to eat, or that my sugar was still running high, so I had to wait until it was lower. He would check the kitchen for signs to prove that I was eating and to see if I was telling the truth. I had that covered though. I would take spoons or forks and stick them in food and wipe them off just enough to make it look like I had eaten. I would smear ketchup or peanut butter on a knife and tell him I had just made and ate a sandwich. On the rare occasions that I did eat in front of someone, I would cut my food into tiny pieces and simply push it around the plate to make it look like I was eating and then toss it in the trash taking great care to cover any evidence that I was skipping meals.

Lies, Lies, lies. Lies are the fuels that keep eating disorders alive. The various methods I was using to lose weight had to be hidden or else I would not be able to continue them. Nobody could know what I was doing or they would make me stop. I did not want to stop. Truthfully, I couldn't stop.

I counted every single calorie I put in my mouth, and that is no exaggeration. I found the lowest calorie foods I could find too. Lettuce, grapes, carrots, unsweet tea (lots and lots of tea), and peanut butter and crackers were my favorites. Nothing went in my mouth if I did not know how many calories were in it. I had a calorie counter book I kept in my car. If it was not listed in the book, then it did not go in my mouth. And if it was too many calories, it didn't make it in my body either. I installed a diet and weight app on my cell phone. I memorized the calories in each of the foods I ate. And I counted. And I counted. And I counted. Over and over and over again. I would stare at my plate and count the calories of each food. If it was dinner time, I would recount in my head whatever I had already had that day. I could not go over my limit. I did not have to count very high because I only allowed myself 500 calories a day. But, that was too many calories too. I would have to find a way to get rid of those as well. While the high sugars were helping to burn off some of them, I was sure I was still holding onto too many of them. Even though I was dropping pound after pound, I was still fat. It did not matter how thin I got. The thinner I got the fatter I felt and the fatter I felt meant the less I could eat.

It was not long until I was back in the hospital again. I had done a good job of convincing them AGAIN that I did not know what was going on with my sugars. I told them that my body had just probably been through so much that it was having a hard time getting adjusted. Each hospital visit, I got pumped with fluids and insulin and sent back home. Before I was ever discharged, I was already planning my next dangerous act. One more cycle and then I would stop. However, one more was never enough. I was spiraling down a deadly vortex to an early grave and did not even realize it.

This was getting to be so easy, skipping insulin and skipping meals. I was looking great. People were telling me how great I looked and asking how I was getting so thin. I lied and told them diet and exercise. I needed more though. I needed more ways to lose so I could keep getting thinner. I had never been one who enjoyed throwing up but I was about to become a pro at that as well. When I was a kid, I would fight it if I was sick. But, I was willing to tolerate it if it meant losing more weight. I mean, I did enjoy the taste of certain foods. I had been missing out on some of my favorites because they were "bad" foods. But, if I ate them and then just threw them up, then I could enjoy them without having them affect my weight loss. So, that's what I did. I ate and I threw up. I did this after every meal. If I was at work I would sneak away to the bathroom after lunch and purge. If I was at home, I would go outside to the back corner of the yard at night and get rid of whatever I had eaten. I excused myself from tables at restaurants and at people's houses to quickly get rid of dinner before it had time to settle.

There were times though when I could not just excuse myself to go to the restroom. So, I kept laxatives in my purse so I could take them now and allow them to work later. If I took enough of them, they made me nauseas later, at a time when it would be convenient to toss what

I had eaten. Again, nothing I did was in moderation. I worked my way up to taking a box at a time. On top of the laxatives, I was also taking high doses of diuretics to get rid of any water weight. All of this was done on top of skipping my insulin and restricting my food intake. All of which I kept hid, at least for a while.

Numbers were driving me crazy. I counted calories in my head all day. I aimed to keep my sugar at least 350 mg/dl or higher. And then, me and the scales got to be good friends. I visited them more and more each day. I woke up and I weighed. I peed and then weighed. I brushed my teeth and then weighed. I ate then I weighed. I threw up and then I weighed. I stepped on them with my clothes on and then would take them all off and weigh again. I leaned forward and then I would lean backward. I weighed at the mall restrooms. I weighed on the scales that were for sale in stores. I had to hit that magic number or else my day was ruined. The magic number, however, never came. When I would hit my goal weight, I would lower that goal by ten more pounds. Just ten more. Then ten more and ten more. No matter how small I got, it was never enough.

If I knew you, your bathroom became my favorite place. I would search people's bathrooms until I found the scales. I would step on and off, on and off, on and off until I got the number exactly where I wanted. If you were related to me, I probably went through your

cabinets stealing laxatives or diuretics also. There were days I resorted to stealing my mother's blood pressure pills because they contained Lasix. Prescription water pills…now that's what I needed!

I did not mean to become a liar and I sure did not mean to lower myself into stealing pills from my mom's medicine cabinet. But, I was hooked. I was an addict. I was addicted to losing weight. As my family and friends began catching on, they began watching me closer and closer. Jason would search my purse and my car for pills. My parents hid their medicines and even their scales. Jason threw our scales away only to discover I had bought a pair to keep in the trunk of my car. He would find a pair, break them and I would go buy more and hide them. I weighed in the driveway and in parking lots only to have him find out. It was not unusual for me to weigh up to thirty or forty times a day. When he would find them and remove them from my possession, I would ransack the house like a junkie hunting for them. I had to know what I weighed. I had to take those pills or else the food I had eaten would stick to my hips like glue I became irate when people would tell me I had a problem. I DID NOT HAVE A PROBLEM. I was just fine. They were all just crazy…not me. I was normal. I was just on a roll with this diet and I felt great.

I was far from normal. I was stricken with guilt with each bite of food I put in my mouth. I would eat just

small bites of meals and then panic at how I was going to get rid of it. At night, I would lie in bed and rub my hip bones to make sure they still stuck out. I tossed and turned because sleep was now out of the question. Every night, I would wake up craving water, and after each glass I would have to go weigh to find out the damage I had done. I would wrap my fingers around my arms to make sure they were still tiny. I measured my waist, my hips, and my thighs daily. When I got ready in the mornings, I would stare at my frail body in the mirror and make sure I could still see every vertebra in my backbone. And even though I could see bones poking through my skin, all I could think was how fat I still was and how much more weight I needed to lose. My cheeks needed to stay suck in. My eyes needed to be hallowed out and dark. That was what skinny looked like. That was what it took to make me feel like a winner. Being a loser was making me win. Looking healthy became a sign of failure and looking malnourished was a sign of strength, at least in my own eyes.

If you could have seen inside my head at that point, you would have seen how it became poisoned with sayings such as “you are worthless. You ate today…that makes you weak. You will never be good enough or thin enough. Only weak people gain their weight back. You are pathetic for thinking you had to have a snack.” I was in the middle of a full blown eating disorder. I was bulimic. I was anorexic. And I also had what at the time was the secret among diabetic women, “diabulimia”—the act of skipping insulin doses to lose weight.

After my many visits to the hospital, I agreed to see a counselor. Actually, I saw two of them and many doctors. But when you are not honest with them, it makes them hard to help you. So I quit going because I did not want their help. I did not want anyone’s help. A friend of mine knew someone who was seeing a psychologist in Jackson. She gave me her number and I held onto it for a while. Just in case.

Finally, one day I hit rock bottom. It was 2:00 am and I was in the bathroom floor sicker than I had ever been. I had taken almost two boxes of laxatives and was staring down a bottle of pain medicine contemplating taking the whole bottle. My sugar was out the roof. I called Jason to come help me get out of the floor and then I called my mom. I needed help. I was going to die if I did not get somewhere soon.

Getting Help

The first step to getting help is to admit you have a problem. I was not quite ready to come clean about everything. I had taken the keys to my life and turned them over to deadly addictions and had let them drive me to the edge of a cliff. There were days I wanted to jump. There were days I wanted to die. I had lost my way. I had lost my faith in God. I had lost my mind. And I was about to lose my life.

I called the number that Tonya had given me and made an appointment with Dr. Willette, a lady psychologist in Jackson. I was still reluctant to go, but when I met her, I liked her immediately. That is saying a lot, because I normally don't warm up to people until after I have known them for a pretty long time. I had trust issues, but for some reason, I trusted this lady. My first appointment was spent telling her about me being diabetic and how everything had always had to be perfect in my life. Be the perfect child. Be the perfect diabetic. Be the perfect wife. Be the perfect mom. She and I both agreed that it was me who was forcing myself to live up to these insane expectations and not everyone else. Aiming to be perfect had indeed drove me to put so much focus on my weight, that it was killing me rather than helping me.

We did not talk in great length about my addiction to dieting at this visit. She did however get me an appointment with a medical doctor who specialized in eating disorders. Before we could go any further, we had to make sure I was in no immediate physical danger.

I was not looking forward to visiting yet another doctor to discuss how to get me well. It would be very hard to fool this one because she already knew my background. I had signed a waiver saying that my condition could be discussed back and forth between her and Dr. Willette. I was going to have to step up my game yet again if I was going to continue my complicated method of weight loss.

At my first visit, the nurse called me back and had me step onto the scales. Great! This was the best news I had heard all morning, a free ride on the scales. It did not matter that I had already weighed close to twenty times already that morning. I was going to get to see if these showed me thinner or heavier than I was earlier in the day. "Turn around and close your eyes," the nurse instructed me. "Excuse me??" I questioned the reason for my not being able to look. "You can't look. When we weigh you, you will not be able to look. It will help you in the long run." Needless to say this did not set well at all with me. I had not been there five minutes yet and already I was ready to go. What kind of doctor

doesn't let you see your weight? The kind who is interested in your well-being, I would later find out

For several weeks, I kept seeing my new medical doctor and my therapist. Despite the progress I was making in admitting my problems to Dr. Willette, I still was unable to overcome the horrible illness that had not only taken over my body, but my mind. On top of the diabulimia, the throwing up, the laxatives, and the diuretics I had been using, I also became addicted to ephedrine, otherwise known as "yellow jackets" or legalized "speed."

I was exhausted from the lack of food, from the high sugars and the constant battle in my head and the only way to make it through the day was to take something that would give me energy. I had seen the "yellow jackets" at the gas station and thought I would give them a try. The first pack I took gave me this incredible burst of energy that left me bouncing off the walls. I was unstoppable, full of energy and talking ninety to nothing. I was hooked. Plus, they curbed any cravings or hunger that I had. I quickly added them to my daily regimen. I started taking two a day, then three a day. Soon, I was up to three at a time and twice a day. My heart raced when I took them. But, when they began to wear off, a sickness would come over me like I had never experienced before. I had to keep taking them to avoid the "coming down" effect. I would come home from work and have to lie down to get my

heart to slow down. There was one instance where I clocked my pulse at 165 beats per minute. I locked myself in my bedroom in a panic trying to reduce the speed in which it was beating. There was no way I was going to admit to Jason that I was hooked on these pills too. He would kill me. That is if the ephedrine didn't do the job first.

During this time, it was odd that the weight I had been so proud of losing, I was now trying to hide. If I was going to keep getting thinner I was going to have to cover up how much I was losing or else I would not be able to continue hiding it from people. I wore loose clothes to hide how small I was becoming. I wanted so badly to be able to enjoy my weight, but I couldn't. I had to keep everything hid. But, I could not hide the fact that my hair was coming out or that my eyes were dark and sinking deeper and deeper into my skull. I could not hide that I was angry and irrational all of the time.

People were trying to help me, and people were trying to hurt me all at the same time. There were people who would say things to me like "you're looking rough. How much do you weigh?" I even had a customer stop me in the store and ask me if she made me a cake would I eat it? Waitresses at restaurants commented on how little I ate. My co-workers were concerned. They meant well, but they just did not understand that I was fine. I

would stop I promised them. Just a few more pounds and I swore I would stop.

One day while alone in my office, my boss, Joey Hays, came in and shut the door. "I would like to talk to you," he said. The first thought that entered my mind was that he was going to let me go from my job. I had missed a lot of work due to hospitalizations and I was certain he was going to tell me that he could not depend on me anymore even though I operated like a robot and could do my job in my sleep. "Amy, I want you to know that I appreciate all you do. And, I'm not concerned about you missing the amount of work that you have. I'm concerned about you living." I let those words sink in for just a moment as Joey continued, "I don't know if you realize it or not, but these folks you work with think a lot of you. They are concerned and I am concerned. I want you to know that we want you to do whatever it takes to help get you well again." I assured Joey that I was fine. I had gotten good at convincing myself of that and thought I was doing pretty well at convincing others too. I told him I was going to counseling and I was going to get better. I promised. After all, it was just anothere lie. After the hundreds I had told, what difference would one more make?

Finally, one morning while weighing, I became extremely excited that I had finally hit my goal weight. I stumbled onto the scale, nearly tipping over from exhaustion, and weighed just a little over 100 lbs. At

first, I was thrilled. But, I did not have the energy to celebrate my newly reached goal. Later that day, I entered the hospital in DKA again. This time, I had to be carried around in a wheelchair because I was too weak to walk. And this time, I was admitted to the 10th floor, the crazy floor as it was referred to among people in the hospital. I listened to a lady down the hall scream and moan all night begging for help to get her out of there. I wondered if I was indeed going crazy myself. Had I reached a point where I could not be helped?

I stayed my normal three days getting pumped with fluids and insulin and going through tests to make sure my heart was going to be ok. I signed off on all the discharge papers promising I would follow up and continue to visit my therapist, which I did. But, boy did she have a surprise for me on my next visit.

SHE KNEW MY SECRETS

When I went back for my next visit with Dr. Willette, she had called in a therapist who specialized in eating disorders. When she brought her in, I was amazed at what she knew that I had never even told anyone. She introduced herself and told me she was there to help me not to hurt me and not to judge me. She explained that she dealt with people who suffered with eating disorders and that she thought she could help me if I was willing to listen. She had already been warned that I was stubborn and hard headed, but she hoped that I would talk with her and then listen to her recommendations. With a roll of my eyes and a nod of my head, I reluctantly agreed.

Instantly I put on my defensive armor and prepared for an attack. I first told her that I was fine. I told her that while I knew I had "gone a little overboard" I could stop when I was ready. She listened to me plead my "I'm not crazy" case. Then she began to ask me a few questions. Though not word for word, following is somewhat how the conversation went:

Therapist: "So, tell me. How long have you been cutting back on your insulin?"

Me: "About a year and a half"

Therapist: "And tell me, how long have you been throwing up outside in your back yard so nobody will know?"

Me: (thinking to myself: "how did she know that?")

Before I could answer she continued:

"How many times do you weigh each day? How often do you feel of your hip bones as you lay in bed? Making sure you can still feel them and not an ounce of fat? How many laxatives do you take a day? Are you weighing up to 30 times a day or more? How much guilt do you feel after eating? Or how guilty do you feel when you don't have the energy to exercise? How often are you lying to others? To yourself?"

I sat with my mouth wide opened in shock. She had me pegged. She knew every one of my secrets and nobody had even told her.

She continued to tell me that I had the classic symptoms of someone with an eating disorder. She then began to warn me what would happen, would not could, if I did not get treatment.

"It may not be the next time or the time after that, or even after that. But soon, when you go to throw up again, to get rid of the food you have eaten; your heart will just stop. Each time you try to throw up you are putting a strain on your heart. And it will eventually wear your heart out and it will just stop." She told me about a girl who had just recently died from a heart attack. She was bulimic and had gone to throw up when her heart quit instantly due to the strain she was placing on it. If she was trying to scare me it was working, at least temporarily.

"So, Why are you trying to kill yourself?" she asked. Now wait a minute? I never said I was trying to kill myself. I told her, "Well, I would not say I am trying to kill myself. I mean if I was going to do that then I would just put a gun to my head or overdose on something." It was not like I had taken a blade to my wrist or anything.

Her response came quickly. "Have you ever heard of slow suicide? That is what you are doing. You are slowly killing yourself. It might take months or it might take years or it may even happen this week. It may be the one thing you succeed at without even knowing you are trying."

She continued to discuss with me how warped my perception of reality had become. She gave me a 6 foot long telephone cord and asked me to make a circle

showing her how big around I thought my waist was. When I showed her, she was stunned at how far off my perception was from reality. When she measured my actual waist I had guessed it to be twenty-four inches GREATER than what it actually measured. "Your measuring tape is not right," I told her. "There is no way I am that skinny." So, we measured again and got the same results. With all of this being said, we began discussing what would be my next course of treatment...rehab.

Rehab? I definitely did not need to go to a rehab facility I insisted. I mean that was for people who were really bad and really skinny. I told her that people would laugh at me because I was too fat to go to rehab. I mean that was for people who weighed like 70 pounds. Rehab was for troubled teenage girls and I was a grown woman with a child and husband. I was not rehab material.

She proceeded to tell me about a place in Texas where I could go for a week long intensive treatment program. She insisted that it was ideal for mothers since I had already told her there was no way I was leaving my child for a stint in rehab. She had a very convincing argument. "You can leave her for a week now. Or you can leave her for the grave later. It's your choice."

I took the pamphlet she gave me and went home to discuss it with Jason and my parents. I was afraid to

leave Haley. I did not want her to forget me if I had to be gone for seven days. She was only 19 months old and I could not stand the idea of being away from her. But, they agreed with the therapist and we made the decision that I would make the journey to Texas to attempt to finally get the help I needed.

SHADES OF HOPE--BUFFALO GAP, TEXAS+

After looking through the information and pondering on whether or not I actually wanted to commit to this treatment, I called and registered for the nearly approaching eating disorder program at a treatment center in Texas. I was going to have to fly from Nashville to Texas all alone. Keep in mind, this was my first time to ever fly! Thinking about it made me incredibly sick, which was fine because that would eventually lead to me throwing up again.

On May 1, 2004, Jason, Haley, and I drove to Nashville to spend a day and night away from home before I was to leave the next day. I was sad. I was scared. I did not want to leave them for seven days. I tried to back out. I thought about not getting on the plane when it was time to board. But, I knew the same reasons I wanted to stay at home were the same reasons I had to get treatment. I had to get better for my family.

We spent the day and night sightseeing in Nashville. That evening after dinner, I snuck away to the bathroom in the restaurant and threw up everything I had just eaten. I suppose I felt it necessary to get that in just one more time. I had to be at the airport at 4:30 am, so we checked into our hotel and spent some family time just talking and watching movies. I held onto Haley for dear life as she slept. Thoughts were racing through my head the entire night. What if my plane crashed? What if I got out there and they tried to keep me longer than just one week? What if Jason and Haley had a wreck going home? What if she got sick? What if she forgot me while I was away? My nerves were a frazzled mess.

Usually "firsts" of anything are pretty memorable, and my first airplane ride proved to be also. When I got to my gate, there was a man there whose luggage was being searched. After the events of 9/11, I did not trust anyone in the airport. Security personnel were tearing his bags apart as they pulled out at least half a dozen cell phones from his carry-on luggage. I am sure I was not the only one wondering who in the world he needed to be communicating with on so many phones. I instantly assumed he was a terrorist and the phones were his way of communicating with his evil cohorts. His phones were confiscated and he was allowed to board the plane…right behind me.

My boss, Joey, flew all the time. A few days before leaving, I was discussing my lack of enthusiasm about my upcoming flight. He reassured me that not near as many planes crash as do cars. "You will know when it's time to worry when you see the flight attendant get nervous. When she stops passing out snacks and sits down, then you can panic," he warned. I thought about that about halfway through the flight. So far, everything had been going smoothly. I was enjoying

making a list of things I would like to have from the Sky Mall catalog as the flight attendant poured me a Diet Coke. Suddenly, we hit turbulence. I watched as she quickly pushed the snack cart to the front of the plane. She pulled down the microphone and instructed the passengers to buckle up and close the overhead compartments. We were experiencing some rough flying and would need to be seated. She then sat down herself and buckled up. Joey's words of advice came rushing back through my panicky brain. "Oh no!" I whispered to myself. "This is it. We're going down." I then buried my head in my lap and covered my head with my arms. I am sure I looked like an idiot to everyone else But here I was on my first ever flight, on the way to rehab, sitting in front of a man who I was sure was going to blow us up if the turbulence did not end it for us first, and now, the stewardess had sat down. My world was coming to an end!

Luckily, we landed in Dallas safely. I boarded my second plane to Abilene, Texas where I was met by someone from the treatment center. When I arrived there, I found that I was not the only one headed to the facility. A counselor picked up me and another lady and we were headed to Buffalo Gap, Texas where we would hopefully find ways to heal ourselves from our life threatening obsessive fears.

The grounds of the facility were beautiful. Looking around at the place, where I hoped to receive some

much needed help with my illness, it reminded me somewhat of a small town that would be near a beach. Little cottages with screened in porches and a beautiful garden area were the first places I saw. It seemed so peaceful and tranquil, just the type of place someone who had gone through so much needed to be to get in touch with reality again, to come to terms with the demons they were battling within themselves, and to find hope.

The first step was to get checked in and unpacked. We were not allowed to keep our phones, our make-up, our medicines, or any food in our rooms with us. No contact with the world we had left behind was allowed except for being able to write letters home. My insulin and my meter would have to be kept at the nurse's station where I could be monitored. While I was impressed with the surroundings, I was not happy about having all of my stuff locked up away from me. There was no point in complaining. I could already tell that they meant business.

The center, Shades of Hope, dealt with all types of addictions from eating disorders to alcoholics to even compulsive shoppers. Most of the people who were seeking treatment were there for a six week or longer program. There were eight of us who were there for the week long program. Six of us were from Tennessee, mainly West Tennessee. I was shocked to see that many of the people who were there were my age and older.

One of the reasons I was not eager to go was because I honestly figured that I would be the oldest and heaviest woman there. I was expecting to find a group of 80 lb., 15 year old girls there. After all, I was an adult, and I should have known better than to put my body through what it had been through. I should have been over the need to look thin. I was married with a baby. I should have been acting like a grown up. But, I wasn't acting my age and I was pleasantly surprised to meet people my age and even up to my mom's age there seeking help too. It made me feel a little more relaxed about being there. That is, if there was a way to be relaxed.

The first evening, after dinner was served, we were introduced to the staff. The center had a team that consisted of counselors, a physician, a nurse, and a nutritionist among others. We also got to meet the founder of the facility. She had also battled various types of addictions and had founded this place to help others who were also facing some of the same problems that she had faced.

We went around the room introducing ourselves. Just like high school or college classes at the beginning of the new semester, we had to tell our names, where we were from, and a little about ourselves. I was not excited with this part of the evening and the founder (from this point on I will refer to her as Miss T) picked up on that fairly quickly. After doing my part and grumbling through my introduction, she looked at me, smiled and

said, "Dear, you have beautiful red hair. You remind me of Nichole Kidman with your light skin. And you have a child at home right? Why would you put yourself through everything you have done to your body? It's obvious you do not want to be here. You are going to be somewhat of a hard one to break down, aren't you? You are the diabetic, correct?" I shook my head in agreement. "You know that you are in a much more dangerous spot than anyone else here because of your health. But, I'm going to help you, if you let me."

Next, we were explained what would be expected of us. We would be served three meals and a snack daily. We were to eat every bite that was put before us and not a soul would leave the cafeteria until everyone had abided by this rule. We were to be up and ready for our counseling sessions and were not to be late. We were to use free time to meditate and to rest. We would not be allowed to go back to our rooms alone, but together at the end of the day we would go with our roommates. And, last but not least, when we were in the restroom or in the shower, we would have to count, sing, or talk out loud. The reasoning behind this was you could not throw up your dinner if your mouth was busy talking.

After the meeting, we were allowed to go back to our rooms and get to know our roommates. As I mentioned before, I do not warm up quickly to new people. Most probably thing I am cold and conceited, but that's not really the case. I just don't like to get close to someone

because then you get your feelings involved. And feelings get hurt. And being hurt sucks.

These ladies, however, were easy to get along with though. While we may have had different reasons for our behaviors, we were there for the same reason...to find peace and healing.

I wrote a letter to Jason and Haley that first night telling them that I was afraid they were going to want to keep me longer than a week. I told them that I could not call them until the day we got ready to come home, and that if someone called them asking for permission to let me stay longer for him to tell them thanks, but not thanks! I was ready to come home...now!

TRUST THE PROCESS

Each morning before breakfast, we had to check in with the nurse for medicines and weight checks. Before weighing, we had to empty our pockets and face opposite of the scale display so as not to see the "magical numbers." We had to empty our pockets so we could not "pad the scales" to keep us from looking like we weighed more than we actually did. They had seen patients load their pants' pockets with coins, small bottles of lotions, and other items to give the appearance that they were gaining and therefore getting better. They knew all of the tricks and getting anything over on them was going to be near impossible.

After our morning health checks, we had breakfast and then yoga or a walk. On the first day, we went walking down a trail with some beautiful scenery. We were told to not walk fast as this was not an exercise aimed at helping us lose weight or burn calories, rather it was to help us clear our minds and get in touch with the outdoors. Forget that! I took off walking at a rather fast pace and was immediately called out on my jaunt. "Mrs. Marcle, you need to slow down. We are not racing!"

At around 9:00 am, we began meeting with counselors in groups to start the journey towards getting healthy again. The theme throughout the program was "Trust

the Process." If we were ever going to learn to function normally, we were going to have to learn that it was ok to eat and that eating normally would not cause us to gain weight, but it would allow us to eat and be healthy both mentally and physically.

The counselors explained to us that our eating disorders were addictions, and that addiction is defined as follows:

"When you don't have it, you feel bad; when you have it, you don't feel good."

I could not have described it better myself. Addictions become much like the famous U2 song, "With or Without You." Neither way was a fun way to live. To attempt to help us admit and overcome our addictions, the center wanted us to feel symptoms of withdrawal. As a part of the healing process, we were not allowed caffeine, sugar, salt, or even artificial sweeteners. All foods were natural in an attempt to help get over cravings and such. For me this would mean that by taking my insulin and avoiding sugar, my body would rid itself of the built up ketones and sugar in my body which had come to be "normal" to me. A week without these things was going to be tough to say the least. After all, feeling "good" did not feel good to me anymore.

Another withdrawal I was going to experience was nicotine withdrawals. I had started smoking when I

began trying to lose weight for two reasons. One was to keep me from eating, and the other was to calm my nerves. I never smoked around Haley or at home at all, but mostly only at work. Smoking is hard to hide obviously because of the scent that lingers in your hair and clothes. But, that did not keep me from trying to lie about that as well. When Jason questioned the smoke smell in my clothes, I would lie and blame it on the fact that I shared an office with a smoker. Of course, he knew better and cigarettes became just another item he would search for when he was performing search and seizures of my car.

Cigarettes were not allowed at Shades of Hope. Knowing that I needed to quit, I did not object to having to go without them, until nighttime. At night, I developed a cough that was not only disturbing my sleep but also my roommates as well. I begged for cough medicine. My roommates begged for the nurse to give me cough medicine just so they could sleep. We went as a group trekking across the grounds to the nurse's station hoping she would give me something to stop the cough. But no, she would not. "Coughing is part of breaking yourself from your addiction to nicotine. If you cough hard enough, you will not want to go through it again. And that will help you not to start back again when you get home." Though what she said made sense, it also made me mad. But, she was

right. I quit smoking because I did not dare want to deal with that horrible hacking again.

DEFINING YOURSELF

We spent each day in group therapy because as they put it, hearing other people's stories would help us to know that we were not fighting these battles alone. Also, we would be able to identify possible reasons for our behaviors by seeing similarities in other people. It seemed odd to me, because I felt that by hearing other people's methods of weight loss, it would only give me more ideas on how to keep up the habit.

Each group session began much like the beginning of an Alcoholics Anonymous meeting. We had to introduce ourselves and tell why we were there. While some people did not have a problem with this, I on the other hand did. It was my problem, nobody else's and we already knew why everyone was there, we had eating disorders. What was the point in rehashing this?

We were told that each of us would have our personal "work session." The work session would be a time where we would get up in front of others and discuss our fears, our past, and our hopes for recovery. We would provide feedback to each other in an attempt to help one another. We would also do exercises (not in physical nature of course) to help us identify why we had lost touch with reality and how to regain normality in our lives.

One of our first exercises was frightening to me. We were each given a sheet of butcher paper and asked to outline how we saw the shape of our bodies. "Draw it as you see it," we were told. After we finished, we were to get a partner and have them actually trace our bodies and then compare them to what we had drawn. What if I drew myself smaller than I was and everybody laughed? What if I had gained and was now bigger than I had even imagined? My fears were quickly put to rest. Everyone in the class had drawn themselves much bigger than we actually were. The point of this was to show us that we see ourselves much differently than the world sees us. We see ourselves both physically and mentally different than we actually are. The sad truth was that we believed it. Besides just affecting your physical health, an eating disorder damages your mental health too. The disorder becomes that voice inside your head that tries to convince you that without it you are nothing. You need the eating disorder in order to be powerful. You need it to have a grip on your life that is spinning out of control. These lies become so embedded into your brain that eventually all of reality is lost.

One more exercise I remember very well was very eye opening. We were each given a sheet of paper with sketches of various body sizes ranging from very tiny to very overweight. We had to pick out which we thought best represented how we looked. Then we had to stand

in front of everyone as they marked the one that they thought best matched our frames. . Again, our perception of ourselves was way off from reality. The point of this lesson was to demonstrate how two people can look at the same thing and see two different versions. The sufferers had unrealistic perceptions of themselves while the onlookers saw reality.

Below is what I saw versus what my peers saw

"To men a man is but a mind. Who cares what face he carries or what he wears? But women's body is the woman."

— Ambrose Bierce, American Author
1842 - 1913 —

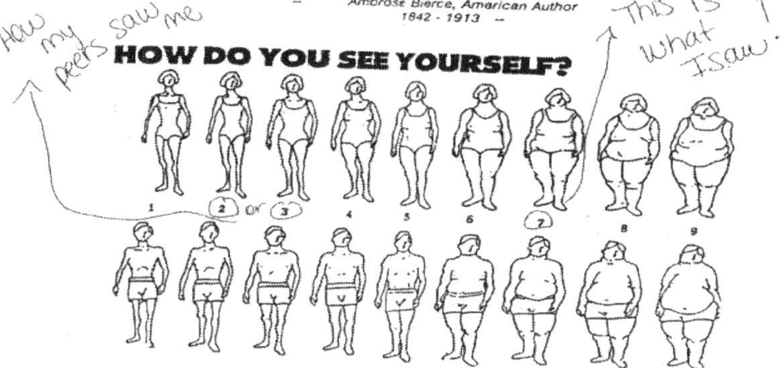

Look at the people above. Then, without thinking about it too much, pick the body that you think:

- *Is closest to what you look like.*
- *Is closest to what you want to look like.*
- *Is the body type that's most attractive to the opposite sex.*

At the University of Pennsylvania, psychologists Paul Rozin and April Fallon tried this test on college students. The student's answers showed that men and women view their own bodies in dramatically different ways.

Men are satisfied with their looks. The average man says his ideal body is number 4 - that's what he'd like to weigh - and he thinks he actually looks like that. He also thinks women are attracted to that type - though women say they are attracted to leaner men.

College women, in contrast, think pounds of fat lie between them and their ideal. They think, on the average, that their bodies are somewhat slimmer then number 4. But, they think men would be most attracted to a number 3 body (when men actually say they like women a little plumper than that). And finally, these women want to be thinner than number 3 standard - significantly thinner than they think would be attractive to men.

- Joel Gurin

As each of us began doing our individual work, we began opening up to each other more. We were watching as strangers were breaking down and confessing secrets they had and the reasons they were suffering. Miss T had a way of tapping into people to make them reach deep within themselves to pull out feelings they had pushed deep inside. I told myself she would have a hard time tapping into me. I refused to feel anything. Opening your heart and soul to feel was also opening it for heartache and disappointment. These were two feelings I could definitely live without.

Miss T had already nailed me from our first encounter when she told me I was going to be a "difficult one." Others in the group had no problem shedding tears in front of others. They had no problem admitting their downfalls, their weaknesses, their addictions. I, on the other hand, was a brick wall, a solid block that you might bump into, but that you sure were not going to be able to break down. I had also built walls around me so high that there was no way anyone could climb over them. I was emotionless, bitter, and cold. And I carried a chip on my shoulder the size of a mountain.

When it came time for me to give my "performance," Miss T had me bring out my tracing I had done of my body on the first day. I hung it on the wall and she gave me a marker and told me to start writing all the emotional highs and lows I could remember from birth up. She wanted me to put more emphasis on the sad

times. Sad? "I don't get sad," I told her. "Write!" she instructed. So, I started by listing things like hating Kindergarten, moving houses, changing churches often, etc. I talked about the day my grandmother had died on the day before Thanksgiving, recalling that I did not shed a tear about her death until Christmas. I told about how I had snuck into my brother, Allen's, room at midnight and told him I could not sleep, because I wondered if Granny Usery was enjoying Christmas in Heaven. I went on to talk about my brother marrying my sister in law, Shawna, and moving away from me; my grandfather dying; a friend getting murdered; and other things I had been through. I relived that day I when my grandfather and Mr. Long had died and how hard that was on me. Finally, I struggled with discussing the details of my near death experiences caused by my eating disorder. Miss T pointed out that even though I was discussing some pretty tragic events, I never cried a tear. Matter of fact, I almost laughed my way through it. When asked why I never showed emotion while talking about these things, I told her "because I have to be the tough one, the one who holds everyone else together." And that was true. When tragedy or sadness hit my family, I felt that I had to be the one to break a joke or make everything ok again. I hated crying and hated to see anyone else cry either. I had always been under the assumption that crying was a sign of weakness, and you could not be weak and keep your life together at the same time.

When I was done, she asked me why I had not mentioned being diagnosed with diabetes. "Because I don't like to think about it," I responded. She told me to describe what had changed in my life since that day. When I got to the part about the doctor who had told me to lose those two pounds, she stopped me. "You are angry with him, aren't you? Matter of fact you are angry about many things." She continued to tell me that she had noticed that anger was the only emotion that I showed. She said that she felt that I refused to admit sadness and concern for anything because I was afraid of getting my feelings hurt or becoming attached to anything that might one day leave me. "Look at all of the loss you have had in your life." I looked up at the names of people on my chart that had either died or left me in some way. "You don't want to feel, because you don't want to lose. And, you have also been in denial about your diabetes, especially, since you stopped taking your insulin. You have pretended for so long that you weren't diabetic that you can't even admit that you are anymore." She handed me two huge, bright red handled pillows and instructed me to beat the chair in front of me. At first, I thought "how stupid?" But, she kept bringing up things that I had listed that had hurt me and the more she talked the madder I got. Finally, I picked up my weapons of destruction and began letting go of fifteen years of anger.

I had seen shows on television before where people who are hypnotized do things entirely out of their character. That's how I felt at the time. Remember the scene from the movie "Christmas Story" where Ralphie finally loses it on the kid on the playground and beats the crap out of him? Well, that was me at the moment. I had forgotten that I was in front of a crowd. I had forgotten that I was in rehab. I had forgotten everything except the things that had caused me to be angry. So, I beat them. I beat the losses I had dealt with. I beat the people who had hurt me. I beat my diabetes. And most of all I beat that condescending doctor who had convinced me that gaining two pounds made me a failure.

I must have gotten too carried away, because finally Miss T pulled me to a chair and set me down. My face was beat red and tears were pouring down my face. My heart was racing and I told her I was not finished. There was plenty more wrath built up inside that I needed to let out. So, I took another round at those poor undeserving chairs. When I finally settled down, I looked around forgetting that I was in front of a group of strangers. Never would I have acted out like that at home or with my friends, but here I was having a meltdown, miles away from my normal life which had become not so normal after all.

I had taken my anger out on everything that had hurt me up until that point. While the situations and people

I was angry with could not feel the thrashing I had just laid upon them, it felt good to let it out. Years of anger and hurt that had been stored in my heart of stone were unleashed that day and for the first time in a long time I felt relieved. "Now, that should make you feel better!" Miss T applauded me. She admitted that she was proud of me for finally "breaking down."

After I calmed down and regrouped, Miss T encouraged me not to let things build up inside of me anymore. "You have to learn that it is ok to feel. It is ok to feel pain, happiness, love, anger. Don't be scared to show emotion when you get back home. Look what keeping it bottled up has done to you." These were things I needed to work on, along with being able to admit to being diabetic. If I could find a way to deal with the issues at hand, I could hopefully lose the need to put myself through the agonizing pain of my eating disorder which had for so long been the one obsession that made me feel in control of my life.

During the week, we had been asked to keep a journal detailing what we had been through with our eating disorder. We also had to write about our feelings each day while we were there. Finally, Friday came and it was the last day of counseling. We had to share our stories and our accomplishments with the group. We then were given our recommendations for further improvements.

I was right about Miss T wanting me to stay an extra six weeks. During my recommendation, she told me that she thought I could benefit from the six week program. She felt I was a danger to myself. Then she told me that she had talked to Jason that morning. He had called to check on me and she said she that while she hesitated in sending me "back into the world," she could see a drastic improvement in just a few days and she felt I would be well taken care of when returning home. I had to write out a plan of action to follow and sign an agreement that I would follow that plan carefully.

When Saturday morning came, I was the most excited person in Texas! I was going home!! Home to my family and my sweet baby girl who I had missed so much. I arrived at Nashville at around 8:30 pm to find Jason, Haley, my parents, Allen, Shawna, and my niece and nephew (Tucker and Ally) to greet me. Haley came toddling towards me wearing the cutest little outfit I had ever seen. Jason had bought it for her while I was gone and she looked beautiful. Her little arms were waving frantically and she was yelling "Mama! Mama!" My fears of her forgetting me had been erased. The best part of it all was that the next day was Mother's Day and we were going to get to enjoy it together.

My family and friends were all proud of me for completing my week long program. I was praised for looking "healthy" for a change. And to be honest, I actually felt good both physically and mentally for the

first time in a long time. It felt good to be able to eat and take my insulin and not be tired all the time. Taking care of myself for just that one week had helped me to break down the barriers that kept driving me back to dieting. But, keeping it up when I was back to my everyday routine would be tough. That would be the real test.

HOME and RELAPSE

Once home, I wanted to forget about everything bad that had happened in the last few years. I did not want to talk about Texas and I did not want to talk about my eating disorder. To me, it was best if I just pretended it never happened. I was going to file it away with the rest of the painful memories I had. After all, I was following my treatment plan and doing better for the time being anyway.

Getting out in public and back to my normal life proved to be a little difficult. People began to compliment me on how "healthy" I looked. While I knew they meant well, my mind was still somewhat twisted. It was hard not to take compliments and make them into negative comments. Following is a comparison of what was often said to me and what I often heard:

Said: "Wow! You look so good. You were looking too thin before."

Heard: "You've gained weight."

Said: "I am so proud of you for taking care of yourself."

Heard: "You are eating again. Why?"

Said: "You look better!"

Hear: "When you said I looked bad, I looked thin. Now, I look better which means I have gained weight. Amy…you are a failure!"

Compliments became misleading to me. If people had told me before that I looked bad when I was actually skinny and now they were telling me I looked good then that could only mean that they had noticed I had gained weight. Something had to be done, and pretty soon I was back to my old tricks again.

Anyone who has ever faced an addiction knows the dangers of relapse. Even a recovered person has temptations they face on a daily basis. Giving in to those temptations is dangerous because of the fear of slipping back into the behaviors you had hoped you had left in your past. While this time, I was unable to lose weight as quickly as I had before, it did not keep me from trying. Visits to the hospital became routine again

and I felt worthless because I had failed at staying healthy.

The dangerous habits that I had hoped to have left behind in Buffalo Gap had found their way back into my life and back into my head. People were disappointed in me for not sticking with my part of my rehab program. My health was soon in danger again. I had given up and surrendered my spirit, my well -being, and my sanity to the eating disorder. Allowing it to tiptoe back into my life had caused me to lose all hope of every being well again.

It did not matter that I was sick every single day of my life. Nothing fazed me. I was going to stay thin or I was going to die trying. Every day I struggled to get out of bed and face the world. Every morning I debated on going to work or going back to sleep. I would wake up and have to lie back down because I was too weak to get dressed. My heart had to work extra hard to keep me alive. Beating harder and faster each day, I often wondered if my next heartbeat would be the last. As scary as this feeling sounds to the average person, it still did not register with me that I was going to die. I was stronger than death. Complications were not a concern. I was indestructible. Jason had begun working as a dialysis technician and came home every single day warning me of what I had to look forward to if I did not stop. Kidney failure, nerve damage, blindness, amputations and the list went on and on of

complications I could suffer from if I did not get my eating disorder and blood sugars under control.

The hardest part of recovery is healing the mind. My mind, my poor mind, was polluted with destructive thoughts. Decisions became impossible to make without seeking approval from someone. If I ate, I would immediately call or text someone and ask if that made me a failure. "I just ate a piece of fruit, do you think I will be ok?" Not only was I driving myself crazy, I was driving everyone else crazy in the process.]

As tired as I was, I could not sleep. Thoughts raced through my head. How many calories had I eaten that day? How many would I have to cut out the next day? The never-ending counting had started again. The weighing, the throwing up, the pills were all back in my life and stronger than ever. It seemed as if treatment was a waste of time and money. I just could not allow myself to be healthy. I had grown so use to feeling bad and that was normal for me. There was no time for sleep anyway. Between the gallons of tea and water I had to drink to keep myself hydrated, and having to go pee every ten minutes, long term sleep was impossible. Besides, I was scared to sleep , afraid I would not wake up. My dreams were the same every night. I had the same recurring nightmare that I was driving off a cliff in a rainstorm and plummeting to my death. That seemed to be the same path I was taking in real life too.

Pushing myself closer and closer to the edge too scared to jump and too scared to be still.

There had to be someone who could help me. Somebody held the key to recovery that would allow me to regain my life. That someone became my daughter, Haley.

HALEY AND HEALING

After many visits back to the hospital, I noticed that Haley was old enough now to start being scared of me. When she would visit the hospital, she would cry and refuse to come into the room. She was three at the time and she knew that mommy was sick. I heard her say it many times. “Mommy sick.” She would say and point at the tubes running out of my arms. At home, I felt guilty for not having the energy to play with her as much as I should. She loved me, and at three years old she was the motivating force I needed to push me to be healthy. I tried hard to hide what I was doing from her. I did not want her to think that happiness came from a number on the scale. But, she would see me step on and off and see me cry in disgust over just a few ounces. And she would say to me “Mommy, you beautiful!” Even at such a young age, she was teaching me more than I could teach her.

One afternoon, Haley and I were riding through Milan when the Martina McBride song “In My Daughter’s Eyes” came on the radio. Though I had heard it many times, this was the first time I actually paid attention to the words. If you have not heard it, it is a song that illustrates how a daughter sees her mother as a hero but how the daughter is actually the influence that drives the mother to be the best she can be. I looked in the backseat at Haley, who was busy twirling ribbons in the

air. Whether she was listening to the words or just by pure coincidence, her timing was perfect. She smiled and said "You are the best mommy ever!" She was unaware that by hearing those words from her at that very moment, she had just provided me with all the motivation I needed to stop trying to kill myself to be thin. I stopped the car and cried. I did not want to be the type of mother who left my child behind in favor of the addictions I had allowed to take over my life. Children imitate what they see, and I was not being a good example to her or to anyone for that matter.

My parents came over a few days later and it was much like an episode of "Intervention" as they joined my little family in my living room and asked what was going to have to be done to get me well again. I never told them about the moment I had with Haley. I did tell them I was ready to stop. I told them I was tired and worn out both mentally and physically.

My body was beginning to have complications from the years of damage I had placed on it from where I had been keeping myself in DKA nearly all the time. My mind just refused to let me take my insulin anymore. I panicked at the thought of what would happen if I allowed myself to be healthy. But, it was time to put this behind me and move forward. My sugar was high, but not really high enough to warrant a visit to the E.R. So, I made a dangerous last effort move to help me begin

what would be my final trip to the hospital for my eating disorder.

I checked my sugar and it was around 350 mg/dl. While this was high, it was not high enough to make me have the vomiting or the labored breathing that usually sent me to the hospital. After all, I had been used to my sugar hitting numbers as high 800 mg/dl. I was going to have to get it higher if I wanted to be admitted. So, I gave myself a shot of glucagon in a dangerous effort to make myself sick enough to go to the hospital. I went to bed, praying that it would not kill me and looking forward to getting to the help I needed the next day.

Sure enough, the next morning I was sick, very sick. I went to work and only stayed about 45 minutes before I called my mom to come take me to the hospital. I was not scared. I knew I was on my way to getting well. When we all got there again, my doctor first told me he was considering a feeding tube and another trip to rehab if I did not learn to cooperate. I assured him there would be no need for that. For some reason, my medical team gave me one more chance to prove I could recover. After a few days, I walked out of that hospital with a brand new attitude. My mind was clear for the first time in a very long time. I was looking forward to living the life that I had missed out on for so long.

REGAINING MY LIFE

If I was going to be healthy, I was going to have to learn to "trust the system." I began re-reading the material I had brought home from rehab. One of the things they had taught us was to say affirmations in the mirror each morning such as "You deserve to be healthy. You are worth the fight. You are a beautiful person." and etc. I began doing these even though at first I felt crazy for talking to myself in the same glass I had used to judge myself so many times before. Convincing myself for so long that I was not worthy to be healthy made it hard to look in my own eyes and find something positive. My confidence level surely needed boosting.

Aside from the physical and mental changes I faced in recovery, I knew I had to rebuild relationships that had been damaged during the past few years. My personality had changed so much during my illness, that people often commented that they never knew which "Amy" they were going to be dealing with from day to day. Would I be pleasant or horribly moody that day? Was I going to be honest or the liar that I had regrettably became? I was going to have to prove that I could be trusted again. And that was going to take a lot of work on my part.

The most important relationship I had to rebuild was my relationship with God. When I say that I put my

weight and eating disorder above everything, that included God and church. I became a totally different person during that time of my life. Growing up in church, I never dreamed there would come a time when I lost the desire to attend services. But, overtaken with my illness, I lost the desire for many things that had always been important to me. Everyone was praying for me, but I uttered very few prayers myself. I was too tired to pray at night and, besides, my mind was preoccupied with my disorder.

During my early stages of recovery, Jason, Haley, and I were lucky to find a church home at Cades Church of Christ. We visited there one Sunday because we were looking for a new congregation to have a fresh start after the hard years we had been through. There we found the most sincere and friendly group of people we had ever met. Haley loved the children and the teachers and soon we called it "home." Jason was soon baptized there and also began doing work with the youth. We had finally found a place where we felt comfortable and loved.

After being in recovery for a few years, I decided I needed to ask for forgiveness for the pain I had caused my family and friends during my battle. I also needed forgiveness for all of the lying I had done and sins I had committed. As I mentioned, I had become someone that nobody really knew anymore. I did not even know who I was myself. My life had gotten so far off track that I

feared I would never find my way back on the right path again. There is not enough room in this book to list all of the lies I told or all of the ways I fell head first into temptation. I knew I had to make things right with God if I was going to find peace in my recovery, and it was at Cades that I felt comfortable enough in doing that. It was a big step for me to go forward and admit that I was wrong. After all, everything I had ever done was done in an attempt to be perfect.

Finding a home at Cades has brought much needed stability to my life at just the right time. We have built many relationships with the people at church and have enjoyed being involved with so many good deeds at this congregation. For the first time in a very long time, I felt that I had found a place where I could belong without being criticized… The people there are not just people I go to church with, they are an extension of our family. Though we are not a very large group of people, we are very closely knit and care for each other greatly. Everyone should be so lucky as to worship God with such a great group of people. For many of them, however, reading this book will be the first they have heard about my destructive past. I hope by telling my story, I have not changed their opinion of me, because friend s like these are hard to find and I would hate to cause them to be disappointed.

TODAY

So, how am I today? Well, I would be lying if I said that I escaped my toxic deeds unharmed. Years of skipping my insulin doses, not eating right, high blood sugars, and purging left me with some lingering complications that I am forced to deal with daily. For several months, I suffered with sore throats from all of the throwing up I had done. My throat was scarred from the acid burns that come with bulimia. I also had blurry vision and many headaches which have gotten better with time.

The most prevalent problem I am forced to endure is nerve pain and poor circulation. A few years ago, I began having shooting pains in my lower back and back of my head. They came from nowhere and were strong enough to bring me to my knees. I visited doctor after doctor and had all types of tests and scans done to determine the cause of this unpleasant distraction. Finally, I was sent to a neurologist who was able to determine the cause of the problem. He explained to me that after all I had put my body through; the nerve endings had become damaged. He went on to say they were much like frayed wires at the ends of my extremities and also in my back. When these nerves touched each other it sent out sparks of pain, much like electricity, throughout the rest of my body. The uncontrolled sugars also led to poor circulation causing me to lose some feeling in my feet. He placed me on medicines to help correct the problem and heal the nerves. He warned me that the medications could cause slight weight gain and asked if I was going to be able to handle that during my recovery. I had no choice. If my nerves did not heal and if my circulation did not improve, I could possibly be looking at amputation down the road. I chose the obvious and have actually been able to come off the medicines for the time being.

The biggest obstacle to overcome when dealing with any type of addiction is the portion that affects one's mental state. Physical damage can most often be corrected and repaired when one seeks treatment. Reprogramming and repairing the mind is a whole different story. I would like to be able to say that recovery is a walk in the park, but it is more of an agonizing work in progress. Though I don't dwell on the numbers on the scale as much as I have in the past, it still crosses my mind every day, many times a day. I still count calories and sadly I still feel an overwhelming sense of guilt when I feel I have eaten something I should not have eaten.

There are days where I want to throw my hands in the air and give up, especially when my sugar does not choose to cooperate. I tend to forget that weight can fluctuate from day to day and often I get frustrated on a "heavier" day. At those times, I admit I have cut my insulin pump off and attempted to get that quick weight loss fix. However, within a few hours I become very ill

and just cannot physically go through with it again. I guess that is a good thing.

Allowing my battle with "diabulimia" and bulimia to overtake my entire life proved hard to recover from. Though it was my worst enemy, it also became my best friend. It was the constant in my life while everything else was changing. By allowing it to be such a big part of who I had become, it has been hard to function without it. Much like when a person loses a spouse and does not know what to do with themselves afterwards, an addict faces the same situation while trying to recover. And, some days it can be hard to resist the temptation to backslide or relapse. Well, it's not just hard, someday it's overwhelming.

People are going to make mistakes, after all we are human. The difference in being a sufferer and being recovered is how I have learned to overcome my mess-ups. I can choose to dwell on them and head back down the deadly road of destruction or I can pick myself up and carry on with my life. It's like I heard my preacher say one time "there is a difference in committing a sin and living in it." That applies to recovery as well. I can have bad days and I can be overcome with temptation from time to time. But, I have to learn from my mistakes and then get back on track. The biggest mistakes made often become the greatest lessons learned.

"Diabulimia" was not discussed very much at all when I began skipping out on my insulin. Matter of fact, for a long time I thought I was the only person in the world who would dare take such a risk. I assumed that all other diabetics realized the complications that could come from such a dangerous move and did not even dream of such a plan to lose weight. I was wrong.

During recovery, I started searching the internet for others who suffered like I did. I was surprised at what I found. I joined two Facebook groups that had been formed in an attempt to promote awareness of this growing concern among diabetic women. Many of these ladies were like me for several reasons. One of which was the frustration that comes with the lack of awareness among the medical field regarding this condition. Only recently has there been much discussion about the need to research the complications and ways to prevent others from practicing diabulimia. In the last few months, there have been articles in diabetic magazines explaining the illness and how it affects so many. If I were to give advice to anyone involved, I would have to break it down in two parts as follows in the next few pages.

ADVICE TO FRIENDS AND FAMILY OF SUFFERERS

As I was writing this book, I was contacted by a young girl via Facebook regarding diabulimia. She had seen a post from me and wanted some advice. She wanted desperately to tell her family that she had been skipping her insulin doses in an attempt to lose weight. Though she had attempted to tell them in the past, she felt misunderstood. Her exact words were "they made me feel stupid." I have never met this girl and probably never will, but my heart ached for her. The most important advice I can give to the friends and family members of sufferers is this: don't blow them off. Many, many times people will take the physical health of their loved ones serious. But, when it comes to discussing mental illness they blow them off as being crazy. When I first began to hint to people that I thought I had a problem, one person said to me "you just want people to think you do. You just want the attention." Heartbroken that someone I trusted would say that to me, I decided not to mention it again for a long time, not until it was almost too late.

As a friend or family member, it is not your place to understand why the ones you care about have the problems they have. Don't question them too much. Don't judge. Don't criticize. Don't push. Just be. Be a friend. Be a listener. Be supportive. Do not say things

to them like "why can't you just be normal?" or "why can't you just eat?" or "why is your sugar so high?" If it was easy for us sufferers to understand our behaviors and avoid them, then we would.

Do not label them either. One thing I have always hated being called was a "bad diabetic." Many people think that because I am now on an insulin pump that it makes be a "bad diabetic." I have been in a room with people who were talking about me as if I was not there and heard them say, "You know she is a bad diabetic. She has to take insulin." When my weight dropped to its lowest, I had a customer ask me one day in the store how much I weighed. I ignored him, but he continued "dang! You are bony. Too skinny!" His girlfriend elbowed him and said "Don't you know she is one of those anorexic bulimic kind? She's scared of food and she is sick." I kept on working, pretending I did not hear them until he finally made eye contact with me and asked if I was one of the kind who threw up after I ate and asked me what my problem was. I looked up at the two of them standing there glaring at me, as they were trying to guess my weight, and politely said, "I sir, do not have a problem. However, I would be more than happy to tell you what I think a few of yours might be." If you must ask about someone's condition, at least use a little common sense.

The best advice I ever received for dealing with people's comments came from Kenneth Ramsey. One day, I had posted as my Facebook status that just because I was on insulin did not mean I was a bad diabetic. After years of hearing it, I wanted to make it public that I indeed was not a "bad" person or a "bad" diabetic. Being labeled as bad at anything did nothing but push me to keep getting thinner and thinner. Being good at losing weight would prove that I was good at something. Mr. Kenneth, who at the time was battling cancer, commented as follows:

> "Don't worry what people say—they need to read Ecclesiastes 3:7—'a time to rend and a time sew—a time to keep silence and a time to speak'—I have had some people that mean well but have said things to me since I have been sick that I sure would not say—I just find more comfort in God. Don't let it get you down."

Mr. Kenneth is no longer with us, but I am reminded of those words often. Choose your words wisely, no matter who you are dealing with, because you never know what battle they are facing. And to those of us who suffer, remember that most of the time, our loved ones who are pressuring us to eat and take care of ourselves are just trying to help. They are just as frustrated as we are.

Though it is important to be supportive, be careful not to enable them with their illness. There is a very fine line between helping and making things worse, and

unfortunately for the sufferer's loved ones, it's not an easy line to spot. As I said earlier, compliments became fuel to my every growing fire of disaster. Telling a person with an eating disorder that they look "good" or "healthy" may seem appropriate but it becomes misconstrued in our minds. Good is bad and bad is good. Try to find ways to encourage them without having to discuss any of their physical attributes. Help them to focus on the positive in their lives outside their health. Point out how well they are doing with jobs, family, hobbies, sports, or anything that does not focus on their disorder. Trust me; compliments are not always the best way to show encouragement.

Realize that our reasons for the dangerous, unreasonable actions go much deeper than a need to just be thin. You have to be willing to help them dig through the cover up that is being used to hide the real problem. An alcoholic will tell you they drink in an effort to "drown" their sorrows and pain. A drug addict may admit to getting high so they won't have to deal with or to feel reality. The same is true with an eating disorder. Controlling our weight becomes a substitute for other issues we cannot control. Never assume that the sufferer is just egotistical and self-centered, after all, we tend to possess the lowest self-esteem of anyone else you have ever met.

Take care not to only choose the words and phrases you use when talking about your loved one, but also be

cautious on how you talk about others. There were many times when I heard people making comments about other people's weight or eating habits and would think to myself "I wonder what they say about me?" When you call a stranger on the street "fat" or make jokes about "how much" someone ate, it causes us to second guess every bite we take. We don't want to be that person on the street that you are making the subject of your jokes. The best practice to use is the never failing adage, "If you can't say something nice, then don't say it at all." Words hurt much worse than stones, so be careful where you throw your rocks.

I consider myself very lucky to have the support and encouragement that I have from my family and friends. It has not always been that easy though. The more someone tried to help me, the more I fought against them. I resented them for trying to run my life and tell me how to take care of myself. Tears have been shed, feelings have been hurt, trust has been lost, and hearts have been broken. If you truly love and care for the person who is bearing the pain of an eating disorder, remember when they say or do things that are hurtful to you, it is not really them anymore. When we get to the point that we hate the world and all that is in it, then we have lost touch with who we are. Be patient. We want things to be good in our lives just as much as you want it for us. Recovery does not happen in a day or a week, or even months. Recovery is a work in

progress. It is a daily struggle that we will be forced to focus on from now on. Stay positive for your wife, your girlfriend, your mom, your daughter, your friend, or whomever it is that you are supporting. Keep hope that the good days will outnumber the not so good ones.

FOR YOU···THE SUFFERER

One song that I related to more than any other during my worst years was Matchbox 20's "Unwell." Any time I was referred to as crazy for putting myself through such torment, I would say "I'm not crazy. I'm just a little unwell." And, that's true. Just because you suffer from an eating disorder does not mean you are crazy. Don't allow yourself or others to make you feel as if you are less of a person because of the issues you are dealing with in your life. Everyone does not deal with problems the same way. We just tend to go to extremes in an attempt to avoid dealing with the feelings we have buried deep in our soul.

In order to receive the help and care you need, you have to be willing to admit and accept that you have a problem. Overcoming denial is crucial. As long as you deny that you have a problem, you are will only be fooling yourself. Trust me...you can only hide your habits and lies for so long before those who are close to you will catch on to your tricks. Remember, if you have to hide your behavior, then you are doing things you should not be doing. Come clean with the people who care about you. Remember, though, chances are they will not understand at first. They need time to deal with your problems too. After all, it affects them also. Once you are in recovery, you will start to realize who your real friends are. They are the ones who stood

beside you and took the emotional beatings from you when you were ill. They are the ones who put up with your lies, your complaining, and your constant mood swings. If they did not love you, they would not have stayed around.

While you should always remember to be considerate of the people in your life, you need to also remember that your life is yours. Don't get so busy attempting to please others that you forget to make yourself happy. If there are people who are trying to bring you down with negative comments about your weight or your life, steer clear of those folks. Instead, surround yourself with the ones who love you for who you are and the way you are. You can break your own heart over and over again in an attempt to impress others, or you can use that same energy to build yourself up and focus on your positive qualities.

During recovery, you are going to have good days, and you are going to have days where you feel like giving up. The hardest day in recovery is still better than the worst day buried in your illness. There is nothing easy about overcoming your fears and worries. After all, your eating disorder has become a part of you, a very dangerous but necessary part of you. Your mind has been convinced that you need "it" to function, to feel alive, to gain that high that being messed up gives you. Feeling normal will take some time, but once you put your past behind you and move forward, you will see

that life is so much better when you can be yourself again.

There were days when I would wake up and be amazed that I had lived through another night. Even now I sometimes wonder why God allowed me to keep living after all the times I had tried to kill myself. The answer is simple. If God keeps waking you in the morning, then He is not finished with you yet. But, you have to be willing to use each day that He gives you to make yourself better. Like my therapist once told me, "your next stunt may be your last stunt." If you have to let go of old habits to get well, then let them go. If you have to lose a few so called "friends" who keep bringing you down, then lose them. Remember, in order to reach higher ground you have to burn the bridges that keep leading you back to the pits. Don't just think about getting the help you need. Go find the help you need. Don't just think about getting better someday. Get better and do it today. "There's thinking about doing something, and then there is just doing it." Regain your life. Find the freedom to be you. And remember, big or little; short or tall; red, yellow, black, or white; everyone deserves to feel beautiful…even you!

FOR HALEY

My sweet little girl,

Well, I guess you are not really so little anymore. You are now ten years old going on eighteen, but regardless your age, you will still be my baby, even when you're ninety-five and I am long gone. When I was your age, I never dreamed in a million years that I would one day have a daughter as loving, smart, funny, and beautiful as you are. Notice I listed beautiful last, not because you are less in beauty than you are in other areas, but because I hope I have taught you that the first three are more important than outward beauty. You have truly been a blessing to your father and I, along with anyone else who knows you. Your kindness towards others and your ability to make people laugh amaze me. The best compliment any parent can receive is one on their child, and I hear those daily about you. I know you have watched Mommy go through so much during your lifetime. You have seen me sick. You have seen me sad. You have seen me angry. I know you have listened to me complain about my weight and my diabetes almost every day. I am sorry if I have placed upon you the belief that the numbers on the scale are more important than the size of your heart. I have listened to you as I have stepped off the scales in tears tell me, "Mommy, you are beautiful, and no matter what I love you!" Those words are what have inspired me to do better, to

focus on the positives in my life, and not be so hard on myself. You are wise beyond your years for realizing what is important and what is not.Just yesterday, you told me we should wear purple for our family picture because you remembered that purple is the color representing "Eating Disorders Awareness." You told me that we should wear it to show we support someone who has been there. That statement amazed me, not because you remembered it, but because you care enough about me to promote it. I will never be the kind of mom who can teach you how to sew or cook. But, I hope that I can teach you how to laugh, how to sing at the top of your lungs to your favorite song, and how to love. I hope that I can teach you that beauty comes from the inside and that is what makes you pretty on the outside. I hope that I can teach you to love and appreciate yourself, even your flaws. And, I hope that you will always know that even with all I went through, I never put you last. I love you to the moon and back a gazillion times!!!

Love you most,

Mom

(3/15/13)

Following is a song I wrote once that sums up how I felt during the worst parts of my eating disorder.

SLOW SUICIDE

Slamming doors

Fist punched walls

Screams and tears down empty halls

My shattered heart lies in pieces

On the cold abandoned floor

And what I feel

Others can't see

New day new mask to cover me

This love has left me ripped to shreds

Down to the core

(Chorus) Cause loving you is slow suicide

A gut wrenching roller coaster ride

Pulling me close to shove me away

Letting me go to beg me to stay

Each day new risks

I can't afford to lose

Live or die it's pick and choose

Slow Suicide

And it's killing me …slow suicide

Craving what's wrong

Needing what's right

Makes for many a sleepless night

It's no longer what I need…but what I want

Can't force myself

To break free

From this spell you've cast on me

Should run like crazy from this pain but I can't

Repeat chorus

(Bridge My heart is breaking

My body aching

Can't find the truth

Blinded by the lies

Can't outrun this

It's you that I'd miss

Cause loving you…

Is slow suicide.

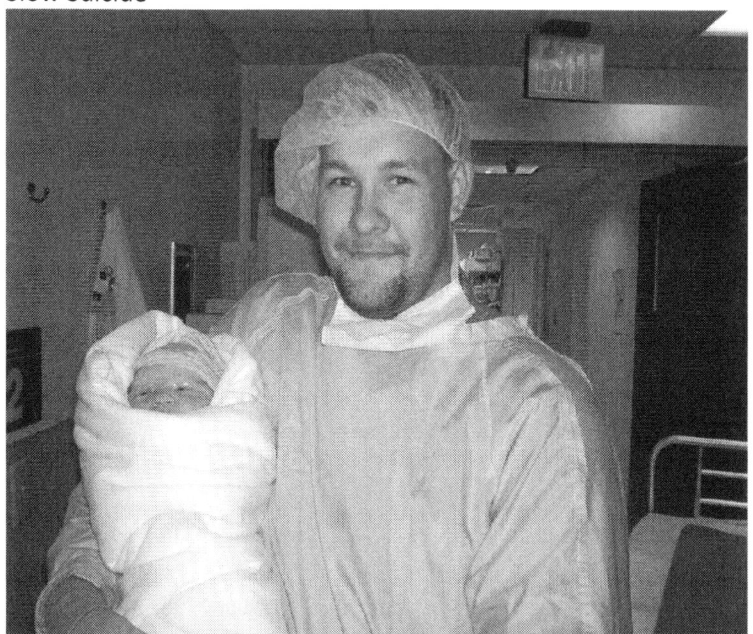

Jason and Haley just minutes after she was born—Oct 29, 2002

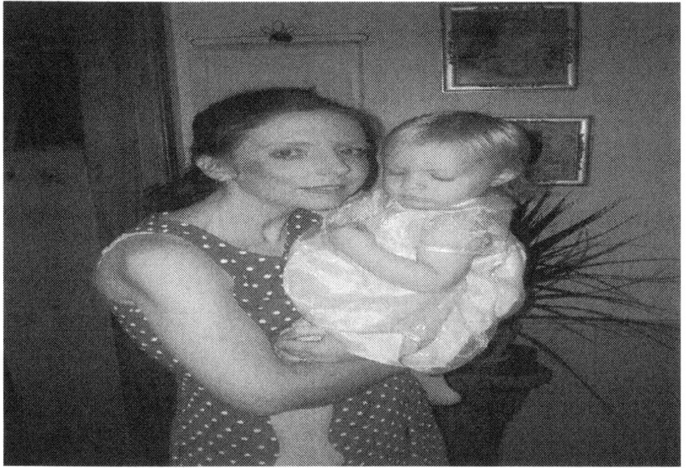

Getting ready for church Spring 2004—last picture I had made before getting real skinny. I dropped 20 more pounds after this photo.

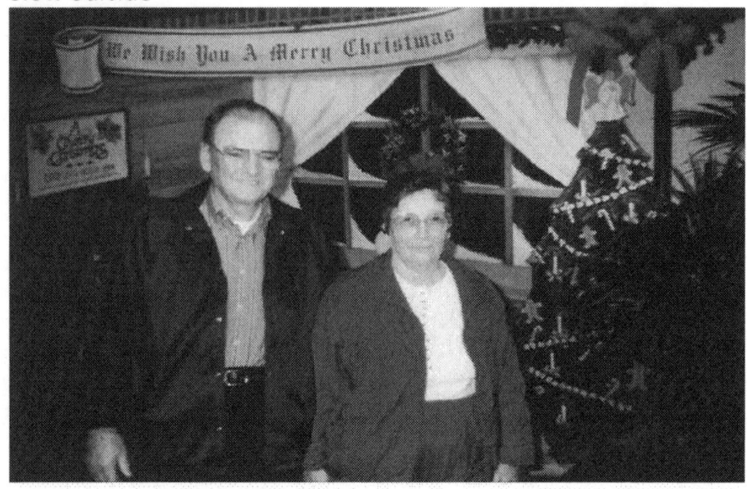

Granddaddy and Granny--Leon and Jewel Pounds

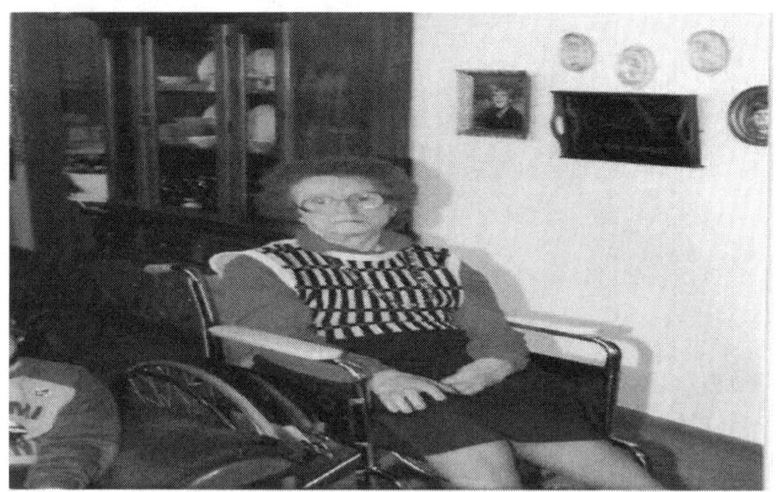

Granny Usery---where I got my red-hair and sassiness to go with it.

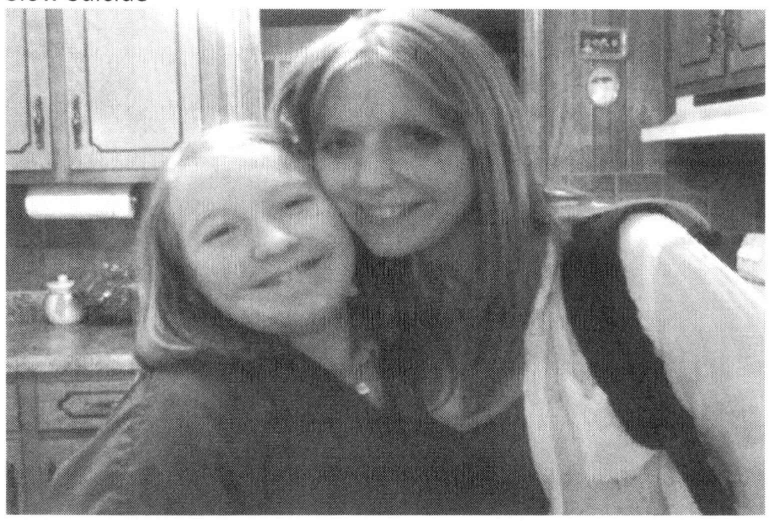

Healthier and Happier –March 2013

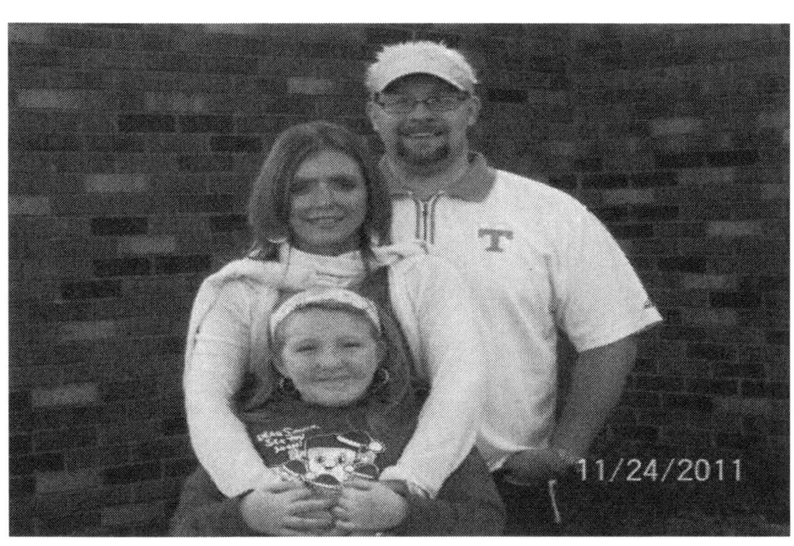

THANKSGIVING 2011 No, that is not his real hair

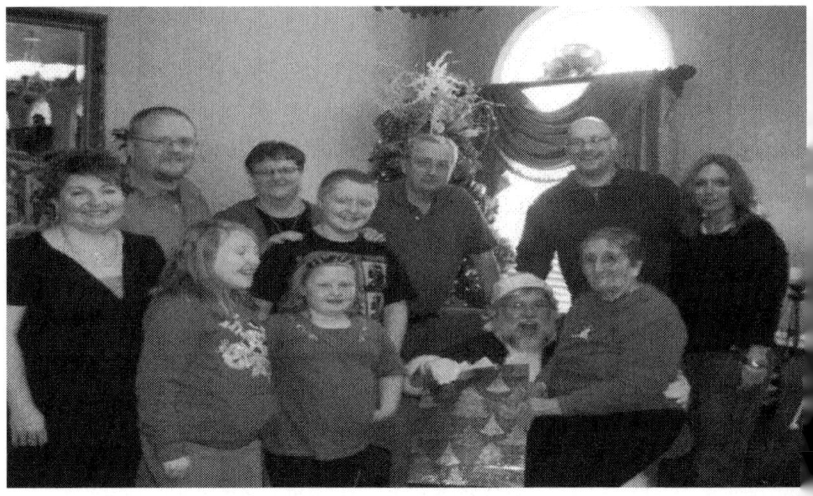

The Pounds Clan—Christmas 2011

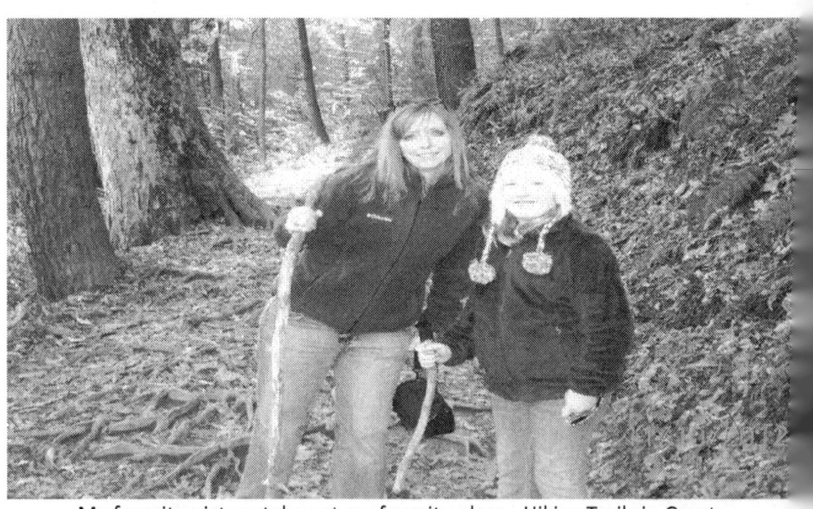

My favorite picture taken at my favorite place...Hiking Trails in Great Smoky Mountains

Inside The Brain Of Disordered Eating

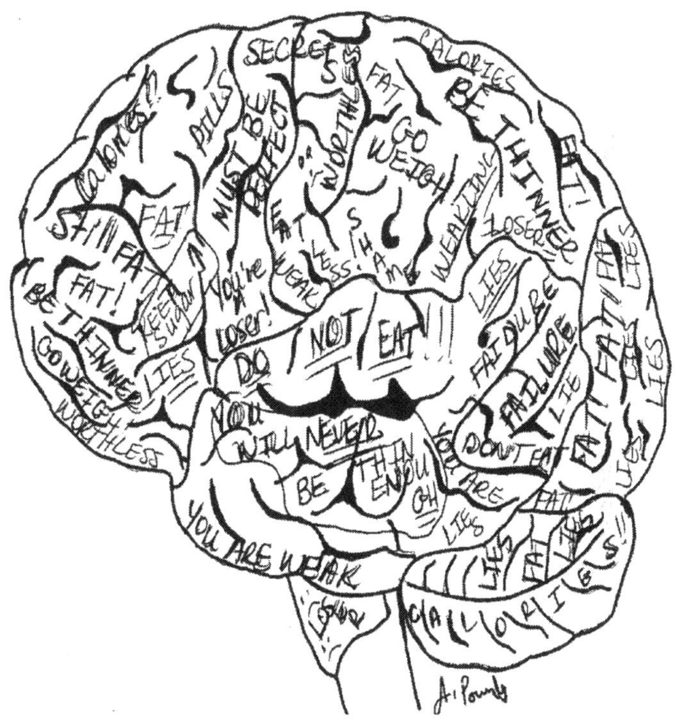

If you could have sliced my head apart, and seen my brain, this is how it would have looked. Notice every thought is negative and related directly to my eating disorder. Did not leave much room for anything

WHERE TO GET HELP:

WWW.DIABULIMIAHELPLINE.ORG

WWW.NIMH.NIH.GOV

WWW.NATIONALEATINGDISORDERS.ORG

WWW.DIABETES.ORG

Printed in Great Britain
by Amazon